I0757216

Accomplished in Verse

Daydreaming of an unrequited love.

A process of beauty and self-reflection that encompasses my thoughts and steals my breath.

A love of peace, an internal sanctuary of balmy breezes and soothing waters.

A rest of the soul and revival of the spirit.

Sprinting, breathless, towards my love of done.

Abandoning fatigue without a glance backward.

Reaching a peak of self-actualization that rains down satisfaction.

Accomplished

How to Sleep Better, Eliminate Burnout, and Execute Goals

Editing by Tamarind Hill Press Editing. www.tamarindhillpress.co.uk

Table of Contents

Dedication

To Harvey and Joelle who supported this book from it's first words to publication. I am eternally grateful for your love and encouragement.

To Zarius, Alena, Sienna and Lexine, my hearts that live outside of my body. You are each my greatest accomplishment and the source of much pride.

To each and every achiever who will read the pages within. You are worthy of every goal you dream. Do more than just dream and you will leave a lasting impact on this world.

Introduction

At 18 years old I was naive and pregnant. The age of adulthood does not always match the age of maturity. Not that maturity would be something one could acquire upon a birthday. Certainly, not in my case. It took me a full decade from that age to acquire an Associate's degree. I think my acquisition of maturity would be debatable even then.

My mother took that 9-month gestational period to remind me daily of my naivety and the gravity of the situation. This grounded me firmly in my independence. Once my son was born, I was his sole caretaker. We co-slept and it took almost three weeks before I relented and asked for help so I could shower. Not the freshest or happiest moments in my life, but certainly the pivotal point.

How exactly did older women manage to have jobs, households, and energy for their children? Did I miss that chapter in the *"What to Expect"* book? How does one manage to recover and go on daily with sleep deprivation? Almost two decades, three additional children and high levels of responsibility later, I have discovered the exact combination required for daily goal accomplishment.

Accomplishment is different from achievement. Achievement is like a 5K run, a small feat that you can check off your to-do list with very little preparation or dedicated time. Accomplishment is the 26-miles marathon you completed after years of training and half-marathons. To reach an accomplishment is to check off a major milestone. Accomplishment is defined as achieving successfully. It requires many achievements to reach an accomplishment.

Achievements are nothing to scoff at. They are the groundwork. The first five pounds you lose on a weight loss journey, the softball game you won that got you closer to the playoffs or making the first sale of a new product launch goal of 6-figures. The small wins increase your motivation and reward your ambition.

There's a reason that this book is called Accomplished. The end goal is to complete a long-standing goal through self-improvement. Empowering you with the tools you need to fuel your initiative to future achievements. The pages that follow are not full of fluff or filler. In fact, I apologize for my brevity. Do not, however, mistake this brevity as an easy path to success. Anything that sounds too good to be true, definitely is. The C.A.R.E method is easy to implement, but a commitment to master.

We live in a fast-paced world, tools that can reasonably fit into a busy day will always win. How you can make the most of these busy days and optimize your energy while grinding towards your accomplishments is the final takeaway. I fell into this knowledge on a personal journey to health that developed into a fulfilling career and revolutionary health for myself, my family, and hundreds of clients.

One part-time job offer changed my entire household. As a dental hygienist, it is difficult to find the perfect office. Corporate dentistry has the lure of good pay and benefits, whereas private dentistry offers better hours and flexibility. I left a corporate office in 2016 and a few months later a pediatric dentist, who also left the same company, reached out to ask if I could work just one day a week. That eventually grew to full time, but along the way, I came across a self-discovery that impacted my health and personal trajectory.

The dentist was passionate and incredibly smart. One look at a person walking in and she could tell what was going on. It was weird talent that I, too, would develop and will share with you later on. Now a mother of four, I struggled with many things in my household, as many others do. However, some carry that in a more personal and private way. During play dates, in casual conversation we omit the persistent bedwetting and night terrors of your ten-year-old, the never-ending antibiotics that are dispensed daily to children that never really get well, or the ADHD that has your oldest child failing middle school. That does not fit into the current social models of today. We share photos and happy quotes to let the world know we are okay, even though we may not truly be.

I knew this dentist needed to see my children. Each one presented with a different struggle but somehow the causative factors were the same. It was a phenomenon that was new to me but became commonplace as I started my own journey to accomplishment. A restricted upper respiratory system can manifest in numerous ways and create a lasting, although sometimes reversible, impact on childhood growth, development, and behavior. A team comprised of both medical and dental professionals tackles these issues to unbelievable results. The dichotomy of this huge unknown field of airway work, that since has grown, sucked me in fast.

I trained and still currently devour all knowledge in this field as a myofunctional therapist. I am the ninja of the team – silent and essential in tackling goals. Years later I can safely say that we have conquered the health issues in my house, and I have aided hundreds of families on their own journeys of personal and physical development. It is in this time of clinical work that I noticed a common thread among my clients: untapped energy and personal drive.

Myofunctional therapy is complicated to understand but simple in its goals. I work with the muscles of the face and oral cavity to achieve proper function and eliminate areas of dysfunction. This has resulted in improvements in physical and mental health, aided in sleep improvement, and created new neuropatterning that changes behavior. All unintentionally.

Regardless of the age of the patient I work with, the outcomes develop similarly. Many of my patients have started out in one place and a few months later are new people. This process I have tweaked and developed over the last few years to adding several dynamic elements that I will share in the pages that follow; to help you achieve your own levels of accomplishment. Before we can tackle them, we must eliminate the barriers that exist to destroy your productivity before it even begins.

There are only two (2) barriers in existence:

- Personal barriers- Any personal reasoning, or lack thereof to prevent forward movement.
- Physical barriers- Any epigenetic result of nature and nurture that prevents forward movement.

Personal Barriers

There are only 24 hours in a day to get things done; an excuse that fails both the sender of that message and the receiver. Consider the use of the word "only." Only is defined as being no more than or solely. Defeat is placed when prefacing a fact to put up your defenses and assemble your troop of excuses. In reality, it's scary to think that only 1440 minutes stand between you and your goals.

The unrelenting feeling of losing control over that time and distance from the goal line becomes a reason to be mindful of this limiting phrase. Control is a concept that we think we have a grasp on. What exactly is within our control and how many things just happen? There may be no real or commonly accepted answer to these questions, which does not leave us with a less daunting possibility.

Acknowledging this absence of answers and focusing more on the goal than the timeframe is the first hurdle to overcome. No goal worth achieving is passive. Take, for example, the dream of many to be a multi-millionaire. There are two ways of going about it and the least passive way still requires work and time. Winning the lottery would require purchasing tickets, checking the numbers (most likely in a repetitive pattern), going to the lottery headquarters of the state, claiming the money, hiring a financial manager, and deciding on future planning such as housing, employment, and vacations. Surely not comprehensive, but very telling that even the fastest route to achievement and satisfaction is not without work.

Personal barriers are comprised of the little voice in your head that focuses on self-sabotage when working on accomplishments. It comes on as a drizzle sometimes and hits hard like a hurricane at other times. This barrier can either be profound and impact you daily, halting your progress in multiple facets of your life; or minimal, and easy to ignore. I suffer from diminished self-limitation. I believe I am overly capable of doing and being anything I want. Typically, I struggle with stopping myself from adding onto my plate or doing 2,874,398 projects at one time. Whereas for others, it may be a struggle to even imagine getting to the next step because those limiting thoughts, statements, and beliefs may be pervasive in your psyche. Balance is important. Learning to acknowledge your truths and silence the objections, while not overestimating your abilities, will be crucial in this process.

No matter where you are on the diverse scale of profound to minimal, these must be addressed or accomplishment will be impacted, delayed, or impossible. Develop your mindset within my C.A.R.E. process in *Section 3*, or individually with many available mindset books, courses, or coaches.

Physical Barriers

For as mysterious and wonderful our minds are, they do have a limit. This is where my studies and daily work has crossed paths with productivity. Ovens, washing machines, and our brains have a self-clean feature. Maintaining the mind at optimal freshness will reward you with fresh cognitive abilities and energy; energy that may have been otherwise locked due to body dysfunction.

Physical barriers consist of the work which is comprised of energy and cognitive skill. This is the greater hurdle to accomplishment.

We currently sit in the timeline of history between the industrial revolution and The Jetsons. Technology has firmly established the hustle and bustle. Balancing family, personal, social, and work commitments is challenging. Often, we neglect the personal in order to make time to satisfy others. This rise in automation has eradicated the necessity of physically demanding careers in lieu of more mentally demanding ones.

Less of us working with our hands and more with our minds. That means the mind has become the ultimate commodity and your most valuable possession. Bodily dysfunction that leads to destructive habits can damage your ability to gain full access to your mind. Functional and fully available make your mind a prime candidate for every task you hope to accomplish. But how exactly does one measure dysfunction?

Through this book, I uncover exactly how to eliminate dysfunction and establish good daily habits that will impact your energy and mental abilities. For many of my clients, whose stories you will see in various case studies, there are even more benefits impacting health and wellness. This book will not, however, be a book full of fluff with no actionable tasks. Even the actionable tasks require some level of effort. Remember, no goal worth achieving is passive.

"Knowing is not enough; we must apply. Willing is not enough; we must do." -Johann Wolfgang von Goethe

Section 1
Prefacing Productivity

Why Productivity?

Every day brings new time and opportunity to get closer to your goals. Every day starts in the morning. Every morning relies on the quality of the night before. Every opportunity is present to a clear mind. Every mind needs to be clean to process new information and form habits. Every habit formed leads to the promise of success.

Let's face it, there is something awe-inspiring about the success of others. Feelings of motivation or irritation develop as we internalize their success.

Success is merely the result of a beautiful collaboration between daily choices and habits formed. Establishing good habits and committing to following through are easy when you have the physical ability to maintain daily energy and motivation. Wealthy entrepreneurs, celebrities, influencers, coaches, or anyone with a platform regarding achievement had to find that balance.

17th-century philosopher René Descartes is famously remembered for, "I think, therefore, I am." A phrase meant to summarize his belief that being is related to having the mental capacity to think about one's own existence. The presence of thought is an indicator of life. The sleeping mind was incapable of conscious thought, yet still important in his theory of life. Yet he had a complicated personal relationship with sleep, being known for sleeping upwards of 10-12 hours daily. He postulated that sleep was meant for the brain to store the information of the day and allow restoration for receiving new information.

Remember that famous public service announcement with the fried egg as the analogy for the brain on drugs? Your brain without quality sleep is like spinach. That bag of fresh bright spinach that overflows in the pan becomes shriveled and small the longer it simmers. Sleep disorders and other destructors of sleep take that supple healthy brain and slowly fry grey matter until your ability to function becomes dependent on a shriveled fraction of what it once was. Grey matter is the brain's composition of neurons to process information. A brain deprived of sleep or oxygen declines in grey matter faster than aging. Oxygenation and sleep are critical to your brain function and overall productive abilities.

Many celebrities discover this the hard way after necessary hospitalizations for exhaustion. When the brain and body are deprived of sleep, it puts the body in distress. There are many consequences that ensue; ranging from poor reaction time to disorientation and paranoia. The most conclusive agreement is that the human body cannot maintain physical or mental abilities at peak performance without sleep. Several studies have been conducted on subjects monitored under sleep deprivation and find that work rates and speed of task performance are greatly affected.

In this way, Descartes was proven correct about sleep. Sleep deprivation will damage the brain's ability to restore and perform. Did more sleep, like Descartes received, in a time where many slept less, give better results? Unfortunately, not regarding health as experts believe Descartes suffered from Delayed Sleep Phase (DSP), a sleep disorder that altered his circadian rhythm. At the age of 53, Descartes succumbed to pneumonia just a few months after starting a new role with a royal family that demanded he adjusted his sleep schedule.

The sun existed to serve as a timekeeper in the 17th century. Many went to bed as the sunset and rose as it raised. The biological clock worked ideally as external stimulants were few and far between. Descartes was a major outlier in society going to bed in the middle of the night and rising midday. DSP did not alter his health directly, however, a sudden change in his schedule did. It is speculated that this shift caused daytime sleepiness resulting in poor mental and physical restoration, which weakened his immunity and shortened his life. In many ways, we have advanced in the four centuries since, and in some ways, we have regressed.

Considering how many Americans presently need to use external sources of stimulation to remain alert and awake throughout the day, along with the National Sleep Foundation's findings that 2/3 of us are sleep deprived, it becomes obvious we are in the midst of a problem. This major problem is not new and traditional methods for improving sleep are abundant. If you limit screen time prior to bed, wind down appropriately, buy just the right mattress and avoid consumption of caffeine or other stimulants within six hours of sleep, you are heading towards a better night of sleep. What if you do all the right things and still suffer from poor sleep?

This question I have pondered for several years. It all began with my oldest child and only son. In kindergarten, the teacher told me that he would be in circle time and as she read a story he would initially be engaged. Then if the sun hit the window just right, a "sun fuzzy" would hijack his attention, immersing him so deeply he would sway his head to match its movements. She was the first person to suggest that he had attention issues. Several teachers later and a rapid failure to progress through fifth grade, the suggestions grew more frequent and urgent. Like many parents, my first thought of ADHD was denial.

We waited the dreaded six months for our appointment with the pediatric neurologist, and she uneventfully confirmed those concerns after one screening. The medication was recommended but the script not filled until our one year follow up. Natural remedies did little to improve his attention or disorganization. Luckily, a few months into the medication, I began working for the pediatric dentist. She was passionate about airway dentistry and made mention several times to sleep apnea being frequently misdiagnosed as ADHD.

Children suffering from sleep apnea, doubtful, I thought. We researched, surprisingly discovering that sleep deprivation in children can be different from adults. Tired adults suffer from fatigue whereas tired children suffer from hyperactivity. My son snored, had restless sleep, and often awoke earlier than everyone. Several times teachers wrote home that he fell asleep in class, which we assumed was due to his early rising. I dove deep into the research and developed relationships with some sleep physicians. Many studies suggest the ADHD is a misdiagnosis of a sleep disorder. They confirmed the connections and immediately diverted from the path of medication to sleep improvement.

We worked independently, from medical providers, as I learned many techniques to improve his breathing and cranial nerve symmetry. Ultimately, things started to improve after we made these changes. Our annual neurology appointment came along in the midst of this work. She pressed on about the importance of using the medication, of which we stopped. I listened, then informed her that we would be taking him for a sleep study instead. That was when it happened, the ultimate disappointment in traditional medicine. She blamed me, without having ever asked about his sleep, and she accused me of not informing her that he even had sleep issues. Time froze and she rambled on about the connection I already was aware existed. I was embarrassed for her. A commoner should not enter her practice and dictate appropriate treatment based on a possible misdiagnosis that resulted in the possible unnecessary medication of a minor. However, it should have been brought up as a possibility or even a question years ago. We never returned for justified reasons.

Whether or not he still has ADHD, as we have not returned for follow-up screening, he certainly is thriving, and his sleep far improved from what it was. The snoring, tossing and turning of before replaced with peaceful, rested sleep. I have a new child as a result. His attention and focus have improved, and I see a drive in him that lacked previously.

In my work with adult clients, I have also monitored a shift. Take, for example, Mary, a 38-year-old female, had a history of braces in her youth, temporomandibular joint (TMJ) discomfort that has increased overtime and currently uses a continuous positive airway pressure (CPAP) machine to sleep. Referred to me by an orthodontist, she visited for a possible third round of braces. Luckily for her, this dentist refused to treat her until she saw a myofunctional therapist. She presented with mouth breathing, crowded teeth, a recessed lower jaw, an open bite, tongue thrust swallow, and no visibility of the throat without manipulation. Her average night of sleep lasted just 3-4 hours and she woke feeling unrested routinely. Her husband died suddenly and unexpectedly in a car accident nine months prior and she had difficulty returning to work. Her psychiatrist was treating her for depression and anxiety; both conditions well managed.

Mary spent 16 weeks doing a dynamic myofunctional therapy program with me. During that time, we worked on orofacial strengthening, cranial nerve symmetry, mindset, and breathwork. Inadvertently, her improved breathing and post-program sleep study resulted in her no longer needing to use her CPAP machine. During the program, she felt a difference in her energy and sought out a new job. Subsequently, three months after working together, I checked in with her to discover that she was on a fast track to a managerial position in her new career.

Mary was inspirational and became more of the norm in my work. What begins with little energy and poor health, transforms into a productive new individual full of life and reaching new potential. The commonality between all these clients was the improved sleep through means that no conventional Google search of sleep tips would provide. It was the beginning of the formula that I find consistently produced the most productivity potential:

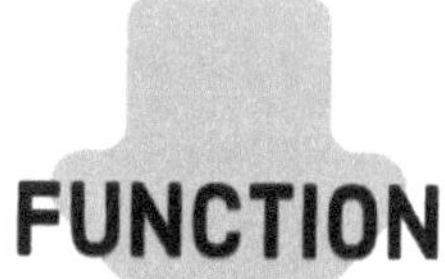

FUNCTION
OPTIMIZED SLEEP
TRUE RESTORATION
= PEAK PRODUCTIVITY

Establishing Productivity

Before we can reach the productivity mountain peak, we have to make our first steps at the base. Psychologist Abraham H. Maslow developed a pyramid theory of motivation. Motivation, by definition, is a general desire or willingness to do something. Maslow's theory was structured to address the various needs of fulfillment required to reach that motivational peak. This hierarchy of human needs has five levels and peaks at self-actualization or peak potential. According to this theory, motivation can only be derived if a linear source of fulfillment is attained. Survival needs preface social and interpersonal needs. A hungry man will not be motivated to achieve anything until the need to eat is met. A man with a full belly and no roof to shelter him will not be motivated beyond achieving security. Once this man achieves a shelter yet lacks human interaction, he will not be motivated to fulfill self-esteem until he achieves a feeling of belonging and love. Only once this man has fully achieved all levels of internal fulfillment can he be moved to self-actualization or meet his full potential.

Mindset and the powerful use of positive beliefs for self-improvement and goal achievement has been recently touted as the way to self-actualization. While ultimately a very effective method of motivation, mindset needs to be supported with other methods for a dynamic outcome. Your brain and heart may be all in, but where is the rest of your body? If there was a steel ball and chain secured to your leg, there would be no amount of mindset tricks that could get you to win a race.

Thoughts and ideas are a great way to support what you can physically accomplish. Understanding the importance of physical capacity as a preface to accomplishment is crucial. At the very base of our existence is a human body with the sole focus of survival. Maslow's hierarchy, in this way, stands as a foundation for the C.A.R.E. method.

Physiological Needs

The inaugural step in our climb to Maslow's mountain peak is the primitive inherent desire for physiological fulfillment. Bare necessities of food, water, and air must be met prior to moving on. Should you have a desire for multiple things and a basic need is unmet, then it stands to reason that it takes priority.

In the reality competition show Survivor, contestants are left in primitive surroundings for 39 days to face various social and physical challenges for a prize of one million dollars. Every applicant turned contestant had a primary motivation for joining the show, many even with sad stories and a desperate need for the prize money. The show leaves them with basic shelter and water, but often the contestants are hungry, living on a possible bowl of rice daily. As the competition goes on, they participate in challenges to win individual security in the competition. As a fan, I can tell you these are some of the best episodes to watch as the host tries to lure them into forgoing their position with basic food. The mere mention of a peanut butter and jelly sandwich can make a contestant forget why they are even competing.

This desire to fulfill the basic need for nutrition becomes in that instance, the dominant need. The brain and the heart competed for dominance and the brain wins. While no contestant is ever in dire levels of starvation, the difference in having three meals a day to less than one is a shock to the system. Food becomes a prize that the mind is willing to work for overall other goals. Pervasive motivation results from physical hunger. Daydreams, fantasies, desires, and thoughts imbed the mind, controlling all the focus until it gets fulfilled. It is difficult to think straight on an empty stomach. Alternatively, what could be clearer than the need to survive long enough to see the grand prize, no matter how large it may be or how desperately essential it may be.

Physiological needs will always trump any other step on this journey. The body needs to be fulfilled internally to reward you with any further productivity, regardless of your goals. Ensure you meet internal needs for the ingestion of food, water, and air daily.

Taking in these basic needs seems easy. However, optimal oxygenation and digestion happen in areas you may not have considered. Improper initiation of these basic processes is like sailing a boat with the anchor down; you will travel but not optimally. Our noses were made for breathing and our mouth for eating. While not many make the mistake of using the nose for eating, mouth breathing will make a direct impact on your oxygenation and digestion. In the next section, I will go in-depth regarding these blockages on your physiological step and prohibit you from peak productivity.

Safety Needs

Scaling the mountain a few steps up, we arrive at our next need: safety. Safety can be fluid and vary between individuals. Some feel security through having a roof over their heads, others may need gates around their community to feel that same level of comfort. Things can create a feeling of security – perhaps a specific item from a loved one or a weapon such as a gun. Safety needs include our next level of desire beyond the physical, the need to exist without external threat.

Internally, there is a conflict that impacts safety as well. You may have heard it called fight or flight. We have a biological safety center, the Autonomic Nervous System (ANS). The brain is designed with one main task, keep the body alive. That is the brain's motivation foundation. The ANS is the brain's connective partner in this task.

The Sympathetic Nervous System (SNS) is sandwiched between the Parasympathetic Nervous System (PNS). The PNS is commonly referred to as our rest and digest system. Stephen Porges, PhD, challenged that idea with the Polyvagal Theory. This separates the ANS into three separate branches of activity comprised of the two separate sections of the PNS, ventral and dorsal, and the solitary SNS.

The top bun of the nerve system sandwich, the ventral branch, is responsible for our ability to actively participate and engage with the world around us. Ideally, we want the body to be primarily in this system. Our neutral is a body in safety that is free to relax. Certainly, not a pina colada by the beach relax, rather a Zen existence relaxation, where without threat we can connect socially.

The bottom bun, the dorsal branch, is responsible for theoretically playing dead. "Immobilization with fear" as Dr. Porges terms it. Unable to engage or flee, this is the option to opt-out. Playing possum and hoping the danger passes or relenting to succumb.

Sympathetic sounds very pleasant for the middle of our sandwich and the third response option, but the name is misleading. The sympathy from this system is only empathic for your imminent danger. Prepared for the possibility of a fight or your flight, the digestive system slows, the pupils and blood vessels dilate, adrenaline pumps, and heart rate rises. With your sight optimal, muscles pumped with ample blood supply and energy high, you can quickly evade danger or sustain a solid grounding in a fight. Either way, the brain is helping you survive whether you want to or not.

The Burning Rooms Analogy

Three men were stuck in a building that caught fire. The fire alarms were engaged rapidly, and emergency systems initiated. In a room, Man 1 assessed his surroundings and called out for help. He remembered basic fire safety protocol and laid low for better visibility. He felt the walls and doors to assess whether it was safe to leave the room.

Man 2, in a separate room, panicked and started to run. He burst through the door in his room and flew down the smoke-filled hallway. He began to cough, and his chest felt heavy. He remembered that there was a window a few feet behind. Catching a short burst of energy, he sprinted to the window and used fallen debris to shatter it. He stepped outside on the ledge and called out for help.

Man 3, in another part of the building, sensed the fire was near. He knew the exits were too far from his current location to reach within reason. He laid down on the floor, face down to cover his nose from the smoke, and awaited help.

Man 1 was engaged in the situation and was led by his ventral PNS. His ability to continue to assess the situation allowed him to process without shutting down or ramping up. Man 2 was in a typical flight or fight SNS response, highly stimulated and full of adrenaline as he attempts to escape. Man 3 disengaged with the situation, led by his dorsal PNS to resist the urge to do anything.

The ANS can be overactive and create this elevated sense of preparedness due to anxiety or panic. Certain triggers from past traumas or childhood memories can stimulate it as well.

I distinctly remember a source of a personal trigger. A typical evening in 2006, my two-year-old son ran in circles around the first floor leaving a trail of crumbs behind every step of his tiny feet. His grandfather must have just finished feeding him dinner and I can hear the chaos below me on the first floor. Baby and I are doing one of our routine exchanges of a clean diaper for the cessation of crying. A brash sound of a car braking firmly on the immediate road alerts my senses mid diaper removal. The house sits on the end of a bend and visibility is usually poor in the evening. It's late and I have little reason to believe that this would be related to me in any way, yet I feel urged by my subconscious to look out of the window.

Part of me did so immediately without thinking and I just knew deep in my gut that my son is out there. Terrified, I move the blinds to the horrible sight of my toddler in the headlights of this car. SNS took over and my feet moved my body fast. I could not process the infant in the crib crying or how this could have occurred. I just knew I needed to move. I burst through the front door, sans shoes or any other practical outerwear for mid-November in the northeast. The driver appeared equally as scared as I, and the toddler was nowhere to be seen. This street was rarely ever quiet, but there was no one besides us two. He points to the backyard and I let my feet guide my body full of adrenaline to the woods in the back.

What exactly would a toddler do when they are outside, cold, alone and likely terrified? I screamed his name into the woods and heard faint crying on the neighbor's wood deck. My heart lifts from its sunken position and I scooped him up into my arms and squeezed tightly. The driver pulled away, I assume, full of relief. His point of escape, a sliding back door, also our point of re-entry, was slightly ajar.

The entire situation was terrifying and highly likely to never occur again once proper measures were in place. Child-proofing ensured it never did happen again. The sliding door he loved being able to open with the lift of a switch, now required three levels of unlocking. He no longer left my eyesight. I obsessed about it for many years.

The sound of a car horn or screeching tire would take me instantly back to that night. Immobilization with activation of the dorsal branch would lock me in my head. Frozen in time, I did not only have a playback of the moments replaying vividly, I'm also paralyzed in fright to the point my heart slows to a near stop and my gaze grows distant.

This is where many of us stop our climb and become stunted on our journey. It becomes counterproductive to have multiple triggers or instability in the ANS. Elevated states of panic and anxiety inhibit the social engagement necessary to complete tasks.

Identifying and reprogramming an overactive ANS requires advanced education and training. A professional team of medical and health professionals is the best approach. In my dynamic myofunctional therapy program, I always start my evaluations and sessions with cranial nerve symmetry.

We have 12 cranial nerves that innervate various bodily tasks. Similarly, to how we must satisfy our needs in order to reach productivity, the cranial nerves fire in order. Each nerve fires bilaterally, or on both sides of the body. The nerve should fire equally and at the same time, therefore, any discrepancies between the left and right sides should be identified and remediated. Without a level of balance and symmetry, the integrity of the unit is compromised.

Cranial nerve X, the Vagus nerve, of which the Polyvagal Theory is based on, serves the great purpose of regulating vital organs. It depends on the function of nine nerves to fire correctly prior to it being stimulated. It is common for someone with an overactive ANS to have multiple cranial nerve asymmetries. Restoring balance is critical in returning to a state of social engagement so that you can overcome and satisfy the safety need. Otherwise, the mind becomes stuck in a state of internal fear, where the brain's alarms are going off and the body is either placed in a state of arrest or hyperactivity.

Josh, a 12-year-old client of mine, was diagnosed with ADHD and high functioning Autism Spectrum Disorder (ASD). His orthodontist recommended braces for his set back mandible, crowded, and misaligned teeth. Mom was a part of a social group of mothers who had experience with alternative appliances and a referring dentist. He was sent to me prior to having his appliance placed for evaluation of his orofacial function and tongue tie. Upon further questioning, I learned that he had trouble breastfeeding as an infant, a thumb-sucking habit until he was five, toss and turned during sleep routinely, and ate food rapidly. During my evaluation, I discovered he had dysfunction or inconsistencies in cranial nerves V, VII, VII, IX, X, XI, and XII. Many tied to dysfunction of his oral and facial musculature, but other cranial nerves had little to do with the orofacial complex.

As stated previously, I start all of my myofunctional work with balancing cranial nerves first. Josh was no exception. In fact, it proved essential as Josh had little attentive focus and cooperation for the first three weeks. He lacked facial expression, eye contact, and an ability to stand still. Social interaction was difficult, and this was expected due to his ASD.

Yet, something interesting happened when we performed a temporary ANS reset exercise. Upon initiation of the ventral PNS, he would look me in my eyes, stand incredibly still and follow direction. His mother was equally as shocked as I, and we made it through the first few weeks of cranial nerve reset. Week 4 we no longer needed to start with Stanley Rosenberg's Basic Exercise. His attention and ability to engage was night and day from our first meeting. Fourteen weeks later, he graduated from myofunctional therapy. His mom reported improved sleep and behavior and progress in his occupational therapy program. The therapy he had for years since he was younger, finally had progress thanks to what I suspect was the shift in his ANS.

We must be able to engage with others and it's not possible if the body is in protective mode due to fear. As babies, we are loved on and given lots of external security and safety from loved ones and objects. Hugs, cuddles, pacifiers, swaddling, kisses, rubs, blankets, and other means of comfort make for great parenting. Beyond those initial infant stages, comfort and security are still pivotal in establishing internal security.

Fig #1 **Cranial Nerves**

NUMBER	NAME	FUNCTION
I	Olfactory	Smell
II	Optic	Vision
III	Oculomotor	Eye Movement and Pupil Reflex
IV	Trochlear	Downward Eye Movement
V	Trigeminal	Face Sensation and Chewing
VI	Abducens	Lateral Eye Movement
VII	Facial	Facial Muscle Movement and Taste
VIII	Vestibulocochlear	Hearing and Balance
IX	Glossopharyngeal	Salivation, Taste and Swallowing
X	Vagus	Organ function, Vasomotor Activity
XI	Accessory	Head, Shoulder and Neck Movement
XII	Hypoglossal	Tongue Movement

Fig #2 **Physiological signs of ANS states**

	Social Engagement	Body regulation Emotion and information acceptance	Calm, Alert, Able to engage with others
	Immobilization	↓Heart Rate and Blood Flow	Withdrawal, Disassociation Shut-down
	Mobilization "Fight or Fright"	↑Heart, Respiration Rates & Blood Pressure	Chaotic thoughts, Poor judgement

Belongingness Needs

True isolation and reclusiveness are rare. We are social beings and our next step on Maslow's mountain to self-actualization is based solely on our needs for love and acceptance. Physiologic and safety needs have been addressed and a new desire for connections now reigns.

A lack of friendship, a partner, or any interpersonal relationships will be felt deeply. This does not mean that having a friend or spouse immediately checks this need off the list. The relationships had should be in positive spaces and leave you with a feeling of real connection. Love, acceptance, value, and joy should result from these relationships.

As you work towards peak productivity, there will be times you desire reassurance, a brief distraction, support, and encouragement. Acknowledge that feeling to have a meaningful connection with your tribe during this journey. You need them as much as they need you. Mutually fulfilling this need helps everyone.

As a baby step towards fulfilling this need for love and connection, try a 7-day personal gratitude challenge. Reach out to loved ones and let them know you value them. Each day pick a new member of your tribe to connect with and extend a message of appreciation. You may not get back the same level of gratitude that you give but acknowledge that this is your journey and your way of sharing your emotions.

I liken it to Aesop's fable of The Lion and The Mouse, where a mouse is spared by a lion and promises to repay him. The lion laughed, mocking the ability of the mouse to help him, a mighty lion. However, the lion found himself caught in a net trap left by a hunter. The lion roared out in rage into the jungle. The mouse, recognizing the lion was in trouble, rushed over to aid him. Immediately, she got to work gnawing away the net from the lion, eventually freeing him. The lion showed empathy in a time the mouse needed it, genuinely expecting the mouse to not be able to reciprocate. Any gratitude given in this 7-day challenge requires no immediate reciprocity. A loved one will return the favor in their own time. This period of gratitude and affection is a personal moment to reflect on who exactly is in your tribe and why you value their presence. Belongingness will come from your generosity in sending love. Taking a minute to write a card, send a text, make a phone call, or visiting a friend, neighbor, family member, coworker or acquaintance can improve those bonds and unveil hidden truths.

Esteem Needs

We are so close to the peak we can see it. The only thing standing in the way is self-esteem. The internal view of self becomes our final hurdle to full potential.

Time to address the little voice in your head telling you that you are not enough, things won't work out, and every other negative thought. Get to know yourself. Really know yourself. Put your thoughts down on paper and address them head-on. Is there truth to these negative thoughts? Would you accept that from an outside source? Does it stand up to measure with the thoughts of your tribe?

Journaling helped me to identify these self-disparaging thoughts and challenge them. I had a low period after the birth of my second child. I spent most of the time with my first-born being very close. We co-slept and did everything together. I was home with him for the first 18 months of his life and had a lot of anxiety knowing there would be a new person coming. Less than a month after he turned two, I gave birth to my daughter.

She was a demanding baby. Contrary to her brother, she hardly slept and wanted to breastfeed all the time. It cut into the time I had available for my son, and combined with sleep deprivation, it caused my postpartum depression to spiral. In my mind, she was born with a mission to tear me away from my son. Every cry and yell specifically designed to control my attention. Within the first few days of coming home from the hospital, it was decided that I would put her up for adoption.

That plan changed, though the thoughts did not after I put her into my bed, and we co-slept as a trio. After a full night of sleep, I put fingers to keys and began to lay out all my feelings into words on the computer. It sounded ridiculous that I really believed a newborn would have evil intentions. I read the words and knew that if anyone told me these things, I would immediately dismiss them.

I did not cure my post-partum depression with the subsequent process of daily journaling, but it initiated the beginning of me being able to bond with the baby I thought I should have loved at first sight. Journaling is cathartic and worthy of attempt when in need of fulfilling personal esteem.

Self-Actualization

Here we stand proudly at the peak of the mountain, overlooking with pride down at our full accomplishment. From this view, nothing is impossible because we have satisfied all our needs and are able to reach our full potential.

Full potential means something different to each individual. Being a better parent, finishing an education milestone, climbing the career ladder, breaking the glass ceiling, advocating for change, or any number of accomplishments. In a state of self-actualization, we are free to explore and actively achieve these goals.

Our body is nourished, safety is felt, our relationships strong with both others and our self; what more could a human being theoretically desire than to arrive at their goals unhindered. In this state, we can truly accomplish anything we put forth an effort to accomplish. Therefore, we have to strive to maintain this state of being by ensuring we maintain our positions at the peak of the mountain.

Lest we forget, where we started our journey had prerequisites. This all begins with fulfilling biological needs that are often silent, disregarded, or ignored. The foundation of which all potential for accomplishment is based has you tethered to the ground, incapable of progress. Your self-actualization may be challenged without your knowledge. In my experience, a poor upper respiratory system in function or structure is the silent culprit of your productivity, as it inhibits your ability to reach true restoration. Put simply, improper breathing is limiting sleep, which in turn is preventing personal progress as two biological requirements are deficient.

Masking it is the falsehood of commonality. Common does not equate to normal. Common is defined as occurring frequently or prevalent, whereas normal is standard or expected. The coworker that comes in and tells you about their long night of poor to no sleep while dragging their feet and sipping on coffee, may be common. Yet nothing about that frequent occurrence is normal.

Snoring and waking tired have established a stronghold on American society. Coffee consumption keeps the body full of caffeinated energy and snoring can be disregarded as we all know someone who does it. Snoring is the sound of air traveling through the airway and hitting an obstruction. It can be a sign of Obstructive Sleep Apnea (OSA), a sleep breathing disorder wherein the structures of the upper airway become blocked and breathing stops occurring frequently. Ten seconds of respiration cessation in these events is the baseline for diagnosis.

Take a break to hold your breath for 10 seconds. Each second will feel longer than the one previous as your brain begins to sense the rise in carbon dioxide and begins to sound the alarms to the ANS. This happens nightly in OSA, several times an hour in some instances. The body jerks awake and gasps for the air it felt the void of. Sleep becomes more fragmented and the brain, cells, and organs that desperately needed the air, weaken.

Imagine a loved one holding that same breath, but unconsciously. The experience is elevated when you witness a spouse, child, parent, or sibling laying too peacefully and not breathing. A mother of a five-years-old client, I will never forget. She cried as she played for me a recording on her phone of her son sleeping while not breathing for eight seconds before waking up violently.

It is estimated that 20% of the population suffers from a sleep breathing disorder. That means that one in five people, reading is likely to never accelerate past the biological need stage. Most are never diagnosed and therefore never treated. In my private practice, I have more clients who come for collaborative services with braces or tongue tie and wind up getting sleep studies at my urging, and the overwhelming majority are diagnosed with a sleep breathing disorder.

This is not something taught or discussed in length in medical and dental schools. Despite a current change in the tides that are increasing awareness, the overwhelming majority of medical professionals are unaware of these links. This is why you may have thought up to this point that you have never heard of this.

For most specialists, it can be considered outside of the scope of practice to look at airway or oral features. When the doctor asks you to say, "Aahh," it is to do a quick exam of your tonsils; not to evaluate the size of the oral cavity and speculate on a narrow airway. Those things are for dentists and otolaryngologists (otherwise known as ear, nose and throat doctors). A referral is the closest you may get to physician confirmation of an airway problem.

"Insufficient sleep is a public health epidemic" -Center for Disease Control

How you sleep matters. It stands to reason that this epidemic sleep deprivation prevents many from accessing their full potential and self-actualization.

I liken this to traffic. The stop and go of a congested highway generate anxiety. Every vehicle has somewhere to go, a final destination. Hyper-focused, many change lanes to no resolve. No one really gets anywhere any faster, we are all just stuck and at the mercy of the highway. There have been no miracle solutions to traffic, especially during rush hour. To avoid it requires a change in the thought process. If you can't be them, avoid them. The innovation of new apps with alternate routes has saved many from the torment of daily traffic patterns. Sleep breathing disorders are the traffic, the merciless warden of the body's prison. You are getting nowhere, especially considering our journey to self-actualization.

We are mere humans and we cannot give what we do not have. Without the restorative properties obtained only through sleep, we are unable to fulfill biological needs and be productive. In the next section, I will give you the knowledge of what barriers to look for and how to begin addressing them. Just like knowing more exercise and a better diet will make us healthier and reduce weight yet does not inherently produce a society of healthier people, this knowledge alone is not enough to produce action. How we apply this knowledge is the difference between looking up at the peak and making the climb.

Lacking the essential 7-8 hours of recommended sleep is not the culprit. The truth is, there is no one size fits all method. Great sleep is personal. What works for you and leaves you waking up feeling refreshed and ready to get through your day accomplished, is sufficient. Your day tomorrow relies entirely on the quality of the night you have prior.

The plethora of sleep tips, tricks, and advice out there may not work. That is okay. Freestyling sleep may not be the best route. You may not be physiologically built to have great sleep. Knowing that you have that hurdle to success is the key to overcoming.

Section 2

Productivity Pitfalls

Blocking Productivity

The first step in solving a problem is being able to identify it. Subconsciously, any barricades to biological needs would have been addressed by the body early on through a compensatory strategy; creating a new level of difficulty to self-identify without training. The things you do and have done for decades possibly may have been improper. While not wrong, because your body did what it needed to do to survive, it was not optimal and may very well be holding you back from reaching that mountain peak of self-actualization. Not all breathing, eating, and sleeping are created equally.

"Failure to identify and remediate dysfunctional behavior will certainly result in relapse." - Roger Price

Breathing is the most essential task of human life. We can go for days without water, weeks without food, yet only mere minutes without oxygen. Without the atmosphere surrounding this planet, life would all but be eradicated. Sleep-disordered breathing (SDB) is sleep affected by the manner of breathing, usually due to an impacted airway. Sleep, when optimized, leads to true restoration, which provides peak productivity ability as discussed in the last section. In my four-step formula for accomplishment through peak productivity, most are missing the first component: function. Lacking the ability, tools, and freedom to breathe unrestricted and under physiologically appropriate conditions, almost always results in SDB. Affecting approximately 60 million Americans and usually going undiagnosed, there are several factors that indicate a higher risk for SDB and resulting sleep disorders:

- Mouth breathing
- Tethered oral tissues (TOTs)
- Improper oral rest posture

Sitting right between the eyes is nature's oxygen optimizing masterpiece. The nose perfects the air we inhale and primes it with moisture, filters out particles, and maximizes nitric oxide. Nitric oxide is an essential compound that helps to dilate the blood vessels thereby increasing blood flow to the brain and body, reducing inflammation, and stimulation of hormone release. When done correctly, nasal breathing can provide health and developmental benefits that are difficult to duplicate.

There are almost no benefits to mouth breathing, as such, it should only be used as a last resort when the nose is congested. Barring a medical disorder or deformity, the nose should be the primary source of air intake. Should you have physical barriers to nasal breathing or difficulty achieving nasal breathing, it is essential that you consult with your primary care physician or an otolaryngologist (ENT) for evaluation. They evaluate and scope the upper respiratory system for blockages. Deviated septum, recessed mandible, enlarged tonsils, and adenoids, among other things can prevent optimal airway function.

Mouth breathing is not always obvious. It can be as discreet as a subtle chronic part in the lips; an unfortunate beauty trend as models tend to own this look in most photos. Sometimes it is as obvious as Napoleon Dynamite's perpetual stance, where the teeth and low tongue are also visible. Alternatively, it is possible to breathe through the nose with the mouth open. Some open mouths are a signal of concentration or awe and not a physical tool for respiration. The long-standing stances are typically the culprits. Physiology can encourage mouth breathing through tethered oral tissues, making it difficult to establish proper breathing.

The human body is a thing of magnificent resilience. The will to survive, and do so by any means, enables to body to adapt to many obstacles. These adaptations can also be interpreted as compensations when it involves an internal dysfunction or restriction. Elimination or absence of compensation is the foundation for a body in optimal function.

The human body is an amazing and intricate work of natural art that we will probably study for centuries to come before we ever establish a complete understanding of it. From what we do know from current research and physiologic understanding, it is all very connected. Every organ, bone, muscle, and tissue are connected in some way to each other. Consider, now, how that connection can impact your goals of peak productivity.

Imagine trying to run a 5K marathon as a three-legged race. The person you are tied to, you have no control over. They are smaller and weaker than you. You may have trained for this race, while your partner has put in little to no effort. Frustrated, you may attempt at some point to carry more of the weight, thereby compensating for their lack of ability to perform. Oral muscle dysfunction will activate the brain's alert system. Compensation for poor functional performance will ensure to help you accomplish any task required by the body.

Carrying an inadequate partner through a race is not a good plan for winning. At best, you hope to reach the finish line. Breathing, as a primary source of life, needs to happen and it's our ultimate finish line. Optimal breathing occurs exclusively through the nose. In our three-legged race to win the 5K in breathing, you need patent nostrils and an open airway, or an equally matched partner. The ill-prepared partner who needs you to output more effort or your Achilles' heel would be mouth breathing, enlarged tonsils or adenoids, a narrow upper airway, or oral restrictions.

Many factors play into how you develop these constraints. Genetics has long been accused of being the reason for a poorly developed airway. Epigenetics, the idea that we are a combination of nature and nurture, is now known to really be responsible for development. We get out what we put into our bodies; therefore, you are much more than the genes you were born with. Diet, environment, and behavioral changes will impact your physical development.

Dr. Weston Price researched the evolution of the human skull over almost a decade in the 1930s. As a dentist observing rampant dental decay in America, he was interested in researching oral health habits around the world. Ultimately, he wound up finding a lack of decay and dental crowding in populations that ate natural diets and poor oral hygiene. Teeth that had never been brushed or flossed somehow needed no treatments. More importantly, were the wide dental arches that lacked the common American problem of needing braces to broaden arches and align crooked teeth. Health was abundant in these populations.

There are many contributory factors in health and development. Their diets and lifestyles may have profoundly impacted their health and immunity. Therefore, Dr. Price's research was not accepted. Two decades later, scientists conducted a study on rhesus monkeys where they plugged the nostrils and forced mouth breathing. This greatly changed the skull and facial development of the monkeys. Long faces, misaligned teeth, narrow dental arches, upper lip elevation, and tongue deformation resulted. If our genetic animal cousins were developing poorly due to mouth breathing, it became evident that the human skull was too evolving.

As society became more industrialized, processed foods were introduced and women joined the workforce. This greatly impacted diets as soft manufactured foods like chicken nuggets and macaroni and cheese took the place of home-cooked meals. Babies were no longer with mothers who could stay home to breastfeed. In addition, the introduction of formula and mass production of bottles, all altered the way infants fed. Many more children are needing braces due to crowded teeth than ever before. Fewer and fewer people can accommodate their wisdom teeth. Our skulls changed and it is becoming harder to ignore.

The tongue is now and will continue to reign as the MVP in oral and facial development. Never to be dethroned by any orthodontist or supplier of braces.

It's a lot to take in; similar to discovering that you lived with Santa and the Tooth Fairy your whole childhood (i.e. they weren't real). How is it that the tongue is so powerful that it has this profound impact on the size of the mouth, the shape of the face, and the structure of your teeth?

WHAT KIND OF BARN IS YOUR MOUTH?

Imagine a simple drawing of a house without a roof. It has a simple three-line open rectangle shape. Two lines that meet at a point would complete the roof and create a pointed top, thus creating an almost pentagonal shape. Now imagine a simple drawing of a barn with a nice rounding that completes the roof. Ideally, we want our palates to develop into a barn shape with a nice arched round roof. Our dental arches should form with a U shape.

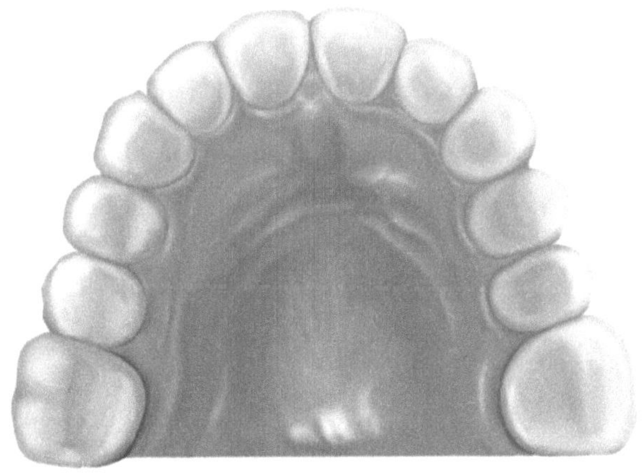

The tongue is the foundation for that development. The tongue should naturally sit up along the palate when we are optimally nasal breathing. The constant pressure of the tongue on the arch facilitates growth around the tongue into that perfect U shape.

Our tongue in that sense is the blueprint for palatal development and should fit in the palate without overlapping the teeth.

When the tongue is low in the mouth, we lose the foundation, and like the open rectangle house, without that round support, the palate forms a narrow and almost pointed "roof" shape. It would create an A shape, narrow arch with a high palatal vault. This narrows the available space for the teeth and causes dental crowding and often malocclusion.

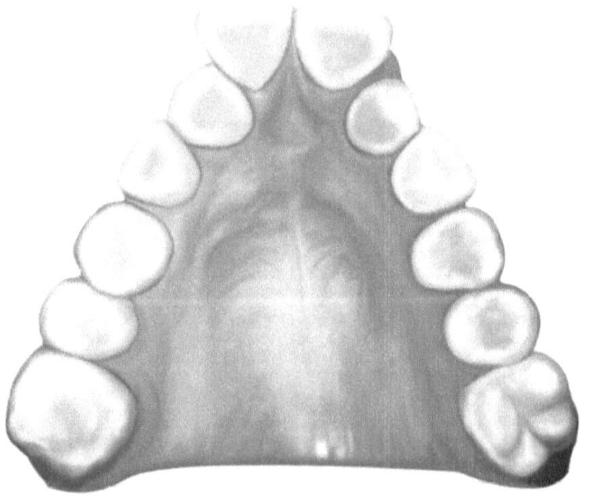

The mandible (lower arch) follows the growth of the maxilla (upper arch). The growth, or lack thereof, in the palate will be matched, in most cases, by the mandible. Those with underbites, or a wider mandible that contains the maxilla (either in part or fully), often have a tongue that is lying low. The pressure from the tongue on the mandible, along with prolonged spacing between the teeth, causes the mandible to extend and restricts the growth of the maxilla further.

What happens, however, when the tongue is unable to reach or sustain elevation to the roof of the mouth? Mouth breathing or an alternative compensatory position has the tongue resting low and against the teeth. With tethered oral tissues, a physical string of tissue inhibits the reach of the tongue up or the lip down.

Lingual, or tongue ties are a common oral restriction that impacts the airway. A tongue-tie may very well be the "biggest little thing" you never knew you had as it impacts and affects many other parts of the body and is involved in an essential bodily function. A connective string of tissue exists from the base of the tongue to the floor of the mouth. We all have one and the mere presence of a strand of tissue under the tongue is not a reason for concern. In some cases, this string can be tight or short which impacts the tongue's range of motion.

Your tongue is like the airport ground crew signaler (that guy on the airport runway that waves the neon wands to direct the plane either into or out of the gate) of the airway plane. Many believe the tongue is a muscle. It actually consists of eight muscles that control the various movements required to breathe, talk, and chew. For purposes of optimizing the airway space, we need to consider the tongue as a respiratory organ. Without the tongue, breathing does not get started efficiently.

The tongue, when connected to the roof of the mouth, signals the Vagus nerve. The Vagus nerve, as you may remember from Section 1, is responsible for fight or flight – the state of social engagement, is the alternative, rest and digest state of function. At rest, in arguably proper oral resting posture, when the tongue sits against the palate, it regulates vagal state. Breathing can be normalized, and nasal breathing, as the roof of the mouth and the floor of the nose activated.

Inability to sustain this position will result in a lower position and can alter the swallow; leaving an impact on the development of the teeth and the patency, or openness, of the airway.

The muscles of the upper respiratory tract relax when we lay down to sleep. The tongue, which can extend down as far as C5 in the vertebrae, needs to be up and out of the way to allow for good airflow. The lax muscles combined with a low tongue narrow the airway and can contribute to snoring and apneas or pauses in breathing – disrupting the sleep and contributing to two unmet biological needs.

10 TONGUE TIE FACTS

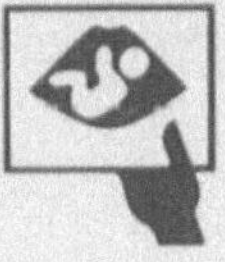

Causative factors can be associated with genetics or incomplete dissolution of the tissue during embryonic development

Average of 3 million cases a year makes this a common occurrence

There are two different types of ties

Anterior - most obvious- tongue is tethered at the tip

Posterior- tongue is tethered at the base

Appearance is not a diagnostic criteria

Obvious tongue ties can be noted by appearance, however function and feel should also be assessed for full diagnosis

Tongue tie can be indicator for a lip tie and vice versa

The frenulum is not a part of the tongue

A tongue tie does not self-resolve, it will not disappear or resorb

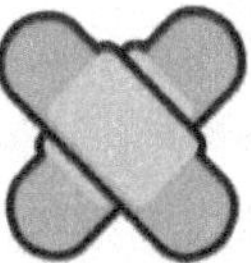

Scar tissue formation can cause improper healing if proper care is not taken post frenectomy

MTHFR genetic mutation is also common with tongue tie

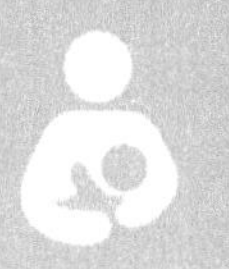

While some babies attain normal tongue function for breastfeeding immediately after release, some may need body work to assist in normal tongue function post-release

"I'm a guy who gets more out of life than some people – more out of one big breath of fresh air than most people get from breathing in and out for a lifetime." -Vince McMahon

Vince McMahon is arguably one of the hardest working men in America. Three other people also stand out for having incredible work ethic: Kevin Hart, Ryan Seacrest, and Oprah Winfrey. With various backgrounds, industries, and ages, there is little to pin down as a commonality between the four. Yet each works multiple jobs, head companies, and major brands, and have families. How is it that they can supernaturally reach peak productivity at high levels and sustain it for decades?

The stamina required to maintain that level of constant activity both mental and physical is high. How exactly does his body not collapse after years of reportedly little to no sleep? Having never met, much less treated them, I theorize that they have strong structural foundations for upper respiratory function that optimize their sleep. True restoration through optimal sleep is the strong foundation for peak productivity. Functioning on full after less than a handful of hours in sleep requires maximizing sleep. In that unconscious state, we are out of control. The only way to ensure the best outcome is to have control over your breathing or having an optimal upper airway.

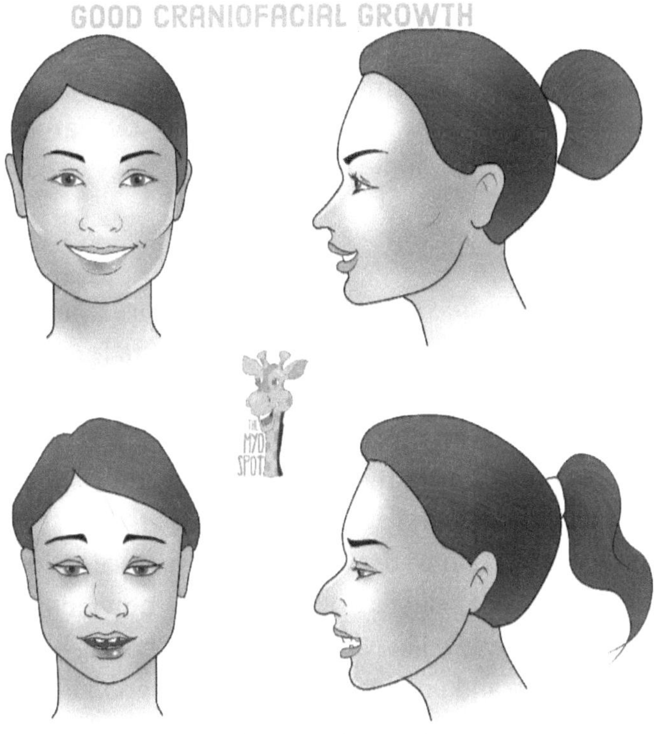

Defined cheekbones, a broad lower jawline with near horizontal angulation, broad nostrils, smooth nasal bridge, and proper head posture are prime characteristics of an optimal airway. Lacking those structures are signs of poor skull development that may have arisen due to various epigenetic factors; putting the body at a higher risk of chronic pain, disorders, or gastrointestinal issues.

Pain	Illness	Gastrointestinal
Head and Neck Pain	Asthma	Acid Reflux
Headaches	Eczema	Aerophagia
TMJ Disorder	Chronic Congestion	Picky Eating
	Middle Ear Infection	

Picturesque model facial features are prime indications that the odds of having a trifecta from figure #4 are low. That is without any medical or dental intervention such as surgery, braces, or dental appliances. Those features are not just physically attractive, they are signs of good function. Recent studies suggest that we may have a physical attraction to those with these features as a primitive way of selecting a mate for reproduction. Not only are they more likely to be healthier, having an optimal wide and unrestricted airway is a good indicator that their sleep is optimal and true restoration more likely.

Mr. McMahon is notorious for never being caught sleeping; a typical success model of being the first one in the building and the last one out. He has personally declared that he sleeps no more than 2-3 hours a night. Kevin Hart has similar sleeping patterns and is fully invested in multiple projects at a time, often working 12-14 hours a day. I dare to say that their 3-4 hours are likely better and more restorative than the 7-8 others strive for.

Oprah Winfrey, unlike the others, openly shares her struggles with sleep and success. Her sleep doctor has made a name for himself promoting the tips and techniques he taught her to optimize her sleep. Her restorative sleep propelled her through the long years of running a production company and doing daytime television. Despite having the structural profile for success, it does not always come naturally. Like Oprah, some have to make life changes to their ideas on sleep and their approach to be as productive and accomplished as possible.

While there are general recommendations for sleep and how long we should sleep, longer sleep has never equated to better sleep. The concept of a standardized amount of sleep was created in the mid-20th century. Outdated and unproven, please disregard the idea that every adult needs six to eight hours of sleep. It is possible to sleep for that long and wake to feel unrested. Inversely, you can sleep less and wake feeling amazing. The quality of the sleep you get is greater than the quantity.

FUNCTION

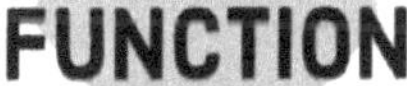

Sleep is a cyclical process where each stage has specific parts that ideally will reset the body. Stage 1 begins the initial relaxation where the body begins to transition from wake to sleep. Stage 1 is that moment when you unexpectedly wake easily from resting your eyes, unaware that you were ever sleeping. It is very light and typically lasts approximately 10 minutes before stage 2 begins for more relaxation. Stage 2 finds the levels of blood pressure and heart rate dropping and the body making an approximate 30-minute transition to recuperation.

Stage 3 is where the magic begins. The body reaches a stage of utmost relaxation and heart rate has reached its low. Muscles and bones begin their recovery, human growth hormone is secreted, cell rejuvenation occurs, and while it is more difficult to wake you during this process, should you wake you will be groggy. Eye movements and vivid dreaming occur in the next stage, REM. Paradoxical, in that muscles become paralyzed however the heart rate and brain activity increases. Your memories are secured in the memory banks and your mood becomes regulated. Theoretically, this stage is when the brain detoxes and uses that self-clean function. Research on mice has shown that cerebrospinal fluid flushes waste from the brain during sleep.

Approximately every ninety minutes, this cycle repeats. Consistency between cycles and times may vary as the night progresses. Occasionally, stages are skipped depending on how exhausted or in demand the brain is for this recovery period. Pharmaceuticals made for sleep or relaxation like Xanax and Benadryl can depress stage 3 and REM sleep. Creating a counterintuitive effect, as the drug should aid in achieving sleep, yet inhibits the restorative stages of sleep.

Frequently skipped or incomprehensive brain cleaning during the restorative stages of sleep will directly impact function, establishing the difference between restorative sleep and rest. It is possible to rest throughout the night and cycle predominantly through the first two stages of sleep with short bursts of stages 3 and REM. The body will wake to feel unrested and that coffee becomes essential to kick start the brain with some caffeine energy. It is not a sustainable plan and will result in burnout and declination of health.

Here is where I believe the Kevin Hart's and Vince McMahon's of the world are correct. They do not need seven to eight hours of recommended sleep. Quantity of sleep is inferior to the quality of sleep. Cycling through restorative sleep stages for long enough to refresh the brain is all that is essential and should be the basis for current sleep recommendations. Their functional abilities with a fraction of the average time most sleep is the basis for my theory that peak productivity is a direct result of having true restoration.

Sleep is individual – the three hours of Mr. McMahon, four of Mr. Hart, and five of mine are all that is required to perform the brain cleansing essential for optimal performance the following day. How much sleep you need is based solely on the quality of your sleep.

Forgo the searching and purchasing of various sleep products. If your body is not designed for optimal oxygenation during sleep, you will continue to struggle with having only rested and never restored. The brain and body will punish you with a lack of performance and your goals will seem perpetually in the distance.

It is time to get on a plan and put the functional formula in action. Take the steps to identify and manage any areas of weakness, start the process of self C.A.R.E. in the next section, and accomplish sleep and goals like never before.

Section 3
Productivity Path

Achieving Productivity

There once was a farmer with a rooster. He loved his rooster, but he also loved sleep. He asked the rooster one evening to please let him sleep in the next morning. The rooster saw the sun rise the next morning and was so happy he started to crow a loud, "cock a doodle doo" on the fence by the house. The farmer, angry to be awakened so early, shooed the rooster away. The farmer decided to make use of the time since he was awake and planted some seeds in the field. That night, he placed the rooster in the chicken coop and asked again for the rooster to let him sleep in. The sun rose and so did the rooster, straight out of the coop to the fence to crow a loud, "cock a doodle doo." The farmer was angry and shooed him away. Reluctantly, the farmer decided to tend to his seedlings and crops. That evening the tired farmer pleaded with the little rooster to please let him sleep in the next day. The next morning the rooster tried to contain himself but was so excited with the rise of the sun he crowed a loud, "cock a doodle do." The farmer tended to his crops but grew increasingly angry with the rooster. He decided to sell the rooster so he could sleep. That evening he went to bed peacefully knowing there would be no loud crowing to wake him. In the quiet of the morning, the farmer slept in that day and the next few. His farm, however, suffered from his lack of tending. It turns out that the annoying little rooster and his habit of crowing at the sunrise served the farmer a good purpose.

The Little Rooster is a classic American tale about the power of consistency and habits. While that rooster may have been frustrating, he inadvertently kept the farmer on a schedule that kept his produce alive. Habits tend to work in that manner, the more consistent they are the more established they become. Habits can either productive on deconstructive. For the farmer waking up early and tending to the farm resulted in great productivity around his farm and yielded good crops. An unstructured change in that habit formed a new neuropatterning that ruined his efficiency.

If you recall back to section 1, philosopher René Descartes had a sudden and unstructured change in his sleeping habits months before his untimely death.

"The best preparation for tomorrow is doing your best today." -H. Jackson Brown Jr.

In the previous sections, we discussed how true restoration is the key to accomplishing more physically and the many factors that may be limiting you from fulfilling the productivity equation. This section is all about how to overcome those challenges.

Function + Optimized Sleep = True Restoration

Translating this equation into personal growth and success involves a process I simplified to C.A.R.E.

Consistency

While ultimately complex, the human body is also very simple in needs. Consistency being the one we thrive on from our first breath and neglect as we let our lives dictate our habits. It is important to reverse the idea that we are a product of our careers or personal schedules. Take it from Ryan Seacrest and Oprah, managing your schedule is critical to achievement.

Upon the birth of a child, the hospital staff will tell you the importance of establishing a schedule for the baby. Babies thrive on routines, they say. When establishing a new life into the harsh reality of being on this side of the womb, it is important to guide them into a sense of structure. This structure will be the foundation upon which they learn proper patterns of eating, sleeping, and play. There is, after all, a time and a place for everything. Do not underestimate this transitional journey you are on. Your key supply along this journey's trail will be consistent.

Similar to the newborn, we need routines in our lives. These daily habits let the body know what to expect and help ease our autonomic nervous system; ultimately satisfying our basic starting ground of survival on Maslow's mountain. We are already pre-programmed with a biological time tracker known as circadian rhythm. This internal clock regulates metabolic processes for the cells in our body. Consistency, with reasonable reliability, gets that circadian rhythm going.

Establish a daily routine for your work and personal life balance but make sure it has a consistent point of completion. End your day at the same time every night and make sure you are in your bed, prepared for sleep, routinely. This sets the stage to alert the brain that you are ready for that transitional state of stage 1 sleep.

It can be challenging if you have small children, travel frequently, or suffer from insomnia to schedule the end of your day. Sleep, as mentioned earlier, is individualized. Be realistic when conceptualizing your new sleep schedule. Midnight is not a bad hour to set if that is the only time you can guarantee you will be in bed. You may be more like Vince McMahon, thereby functioning well on less sleep than average. Wherein time is not the key, as we are not searching for a predetermined number of hours; rather, an optimal quality output of sleep.

I will be the first to admit that my sleep duration is rather inconsistent. It can be very challenging to have an accomplished day and fall asleep at the same hour. The goal is always to be in bed at 10pm. However, regardless of the time I get into bed, or the time I wake as a result, I always am restored. The key is having the ability to remain consistent with the routine prior to getting into the bed.

Your routine may not be perfect every single night. Life happens – kids, family, date night, events, vacations, etc. Things come up that will throw off a routine. The routine should be practical enough that even on a late return or altered evening you can complete some if not all of it without stress.

Establish a nighttime ritual. You may choose a lengthy process of showering, brushing, watching your favorite evening drama, and lay down to fall asleep after the last commercial, or simply just fall into the bed at night. Either way, make it as consistent as possible. You are the baby on the productivity path and need this routine to adapt to your impending new reality. Remain consistent with your routine and your body will reward you with optimal recovery translating to optimal output or productivity.

Airway Optimization

When physical barriers to an optimal airway are present, they should be addressed with an interdisciplinary team. The size of your team may reflect the size of your restrictions. There are many ways to make a large impact with a small team or by working in stages, but the full support of all members is critical to success.

First step is always to rule out sleep apnea or any other potentially detrimental sleep disorders. When possible, ideal care is a sleep study performed in a professional setting monitored by trained staff. The subsequent option is to perform a home sleep study on self-applied and unmonitored equipment, issued by your sleep physician. Our DIY and least desired, though most preferred based on financial restrictions, is self-monitored results from personal devices.

Your primary care physician may immediately disregard your request for a sleep study or referral if based on just self-interest. They are costly tests that insurance prefers not to pay for when there is no basis to do so. Go in with a prefilled sleep screening test such as:

- Epworth Sleepiness Scale
- STOP- BANG Questionnaire
- Berlin Sleep Questionnaire

All of the above can be found in easy to print pdf format on the American Sleep Apnea Association website (www.sleepapnea.org/learn/sleep-apnea/do-i-have-sleep-apnea/four-sleep-apnea-tests-you-can-take-right-now/). A moderate to high-risk score on these assessments can give more claim to your need to have additional medical testing.

Alternatively, a low-risk score may mean you can bypass this step and possibly self-screen safely. Monitor your sleep on a personal device using an app or smartwatch with the capability to assess your heart rate.

Some apps I love, that may help you:

- Oura

- SnoreLab
- Sleepzy
- Sleep Booster
- SleepHealth

Once a sleep disorder has been addressed or ruled out, consider optimizing nasal breathing. Nasal hygiene is equally as important as any other hygiene. The nose is not an inferior body part requiring no maintenance to function. Keep the nostrils patent and available for breathing by cleansing daily. Saline rinses, preferably with Xylitol, help to cleanse the passage and thin out mucus. Xylitol amplifies the help by reducing inflammation. A clean nasal passage always precedes a clear nasal passage.

Prior to starting your saline routine, blow your nose to remove any excess mucus or debris. Equivalently to sweeping the floor prior to mopping, the nostril should be as clear as possible to optimize saline flow. When performing your saline rinse, it is helpful to be nearby a sink or countertop to limit mess. Many rinses have some level of dripping or pouring that will easily create an unexpected mess if not prepared. However, the market is diverse and full of innovation so always use as directed on the packaging.

Getting the nasal passage clean is merely the beginning. An empty pathway is an open pathway. Aromatherapy with essential oils is one of the most reliable holistic health options available. Establishing nasal breathing requires the passages to be decongested and open to the natural flow of air. Oils can be diffused, misted or used directly via a nasal inhaler tube to have the benefits travel through the body via the airway.

Peppermint and eucalyptus oils are commonly used for improving breathing. Peppermint oil decongests, relaxes the muscles of the respiratory tract, and is calming. Combined with eucalyptus oil, which has similar anti-inflammatory and respiratory benefits, it boosts the aromatic effects on the airway. Invigorate your upper airway with these two oils daily.

Lastly, our clean and refreshed nostrils can benefit from uplifting. A physical lift open to broadening the tract through which our air will pass. Nasal strips or dilators can be purchased and used during sleep to reinforce nasal breathing. The nasal strips are single-use adhesive strips applied horizontally over the nasal bridge. It lifts the sides of the nostrils allowing more air to pass. Nasal dilators have little wings that open the nostrils from within.

Some nasal dilators I love that may help you:

- Pronto Sleep
- Breathe Right Strips
- Sleep Right Breathe Aid

Daily airway management should consist of a solid routine of daily nasal hygiene; preferably as a part of your consistent pre-bed routine. However, anytime you can breathe optimally through your nose is a good time. Start slowly to integrate it as a habit. Pick one day of your week initially and commit to performing nasal hygiene at some point during that day. Choose a day that you may get out of work early, have a shorter workload, or are off. As time progresses, you should get more efficient. After a few weeks, add another day to the commitment. Slowly over the course of a few months, you should be well into seven days a week of a proficient nasal hygiene regiment.

"Failure to identify and remediate dysfunctional behavior will certainly result in relapse." -Roger Price

Self-management of the airway can take you far. However, airway is typically a team consisting of an interdisciplinary group of providers. Establishing nasal breathing and elimination of compensatory orofacial dysfunction is the task of the myofunctional therapist of the team.

Myofunctional therapy is often difficult to understand and can be broken down closest to personal training. Imagine needing to strengthen your bicep, however, every time you need to move your bicep your opposite arm is used for support. It would be nearly impossible to strengthen the bicep and difficult to complete any task that requires both arms without contorting the body to compensate. The personal trainer would be working with you to isolate that bicep and establish movements that improve functional ability.

Myofunctional therapists focus on the muscles below the eyes and above the shoulders. Pivotal focus is on establishing proper oral resting posture through tongue strength, isolation, and function. The goals are to establish a tongue against the palate resting posture, lips closed, and predominant nasal breathing. We use various exercises, tools, and activities to accomplish these goals. Similar to working with a personal trainer, these exercises require practice. The trainer is not working with you every day in the gym, but you are still committed to keeping an exercise regimen. Daily sessions of practice and implementing these new movements are required.

Research and studies of this century-old practice have been done in five continents. It has been proven to be a great aid in the treatment of:

- Orthodontic retention (preventing relapse after dental braces come off)
- Sleep Apnea and Sleep Disordered Breathing
- CPAP (continuous positive airway pressure machine) use
- ADHD (Attention Deficit Hyperactivity Disorder) in those misdiagnosed due to SDB

Oral resting posture matters. It impacts how we develop as you can recall from Section 2. Therefore, it impacts overall health and wellness. Resting posture is the predominant amount of time we spend. Every second, minute, and hour that you are not talking, eating, drinking, laughing, or doing anything involving your mouth, you are at rest. Those hours you spend sleeping will make up for any exceptions. Commitment to completing a program is key to establishing a lasting change in oral resting posture.

Myofunctional therapists traditionally are either speech language-pathologists (SLP) or registered dental hygienists (RDH). However, with the expansion of the field, many other health professionals have become trained. No matter the original profession, working 1 to 1 with a trained myofunctional therapist is the most ideal method. I am, alternatively, a firm believer that you can achieve proper oral resting posture through self-taught methods. How you do your self-taught program matters.

Without proper training, you cannot ever know your personal level of dysfunction. Going through YouTube videos randomly to perform exercises does not achieve success. It may, in turn, create a different dysfunction as you can easily overdevelop your musculature. Guided training is preferable. Using a book or professionally created online course with a general program as a basis creates better outcomes. As of the publication of this *"You're Breathing Wrong"* is the only myofunctional therapy self-guided book.

How do you know if you need myofunctional therapy? There are assessments that are available online.

You can download my airway assessment for free at www.themyospot.com/forms. A faster method is my 1-minute breath test.

1-Minute Breath Test

Sit upright in a chair with your feet flat against the floor and take in a deep breath. Notice your mouth during the breath and repeat if necessary. Were your lips sealed? Where was your tongue positioned? Did you feel the breath in your chest?

Repeat the breath, but this time place your tongue up against the roof of the mouth, then inhale and exhale exclusively through the nose. Compare the two breaths.

If your first breath felt more labored than the second, then you're breathing wrong.

In your first breath, you may have used your mouth, had your tongue pressed against your teeth, possibly on the floor of the mouth, or breathed with your chest. Any one of those during frequent breathing is incorrect. Myofunctional therapy would be of the most benefit to you.

It is never too late to acquire the benefits of better breathing. The three goals – tongue up, lips closed, and nasal breathing – can help restore a normal and natural function to the body, and when started early enough can dramatically impact dental arch formation, facial development, and airway patency.

Not all myofunctional therapy is created equally. Various medical and dental professionals can offer this therapy. Some rely on it heavily, while others, like myself, prefer to combine it for a dynamic and more effective treatment. When searching for a therapist, be sure to ask about any supporting methods in treatment. To reach the peak of Maslow's mountain and achieve full potential, we have to work through many layers. Biological and safety needs should be combined in myofunctional services, when possible, to save time and money.

Myofunctional therapy is many things, but a stand-alone treatment, it is not. Even a dynamic provider has a group of like-minded professionals they refer to. A team approach provides the best results when modification of the upper airway is essential. Orthodontic or appliance treatment aids in the expansion of the maxillary arch, speeding up treatment timelines and promoting retention.

Oral appliances are numerous in design and providers. Dentists have appliances that can expand the palate, advance the mandible, inhibit poor habits, or relieve grinding/clenching wear on teeth. Most of those appliances are ideal for therapy – during the use of, some require completion and then starting therapy after to retain or retrain posture. Talk to a myofunctional therapist to get an idea of what providers and appliances they work with. Often, we have an idea of what referral will help you most based on previous client similarities and results. Or work backward and get personal reviews and recommendations from one of our communities on

Facebook. (facebook.com/groups/accomplishedfamily, facebook.com/groups/accomplishedwork, or facebook.com/groups/accomplishedhealth)

Relaxation

There is a process with sequential stages that occur routinely with both earthquakes and sleep. There are subtle changes in the surface of the earth before the actual tremor of the earthquake. During the earthquake, there are rapid changes within and on the earth's surface, and we all must brace ourselves for the aftershock. Prior to our stage 1 transitionary phase, the body is making those subtle changes required for it to fully transition. Your brain needs to have a calm before the storm that is sleep. The body may be paralyzed once you reach REM sleep, however, your brain fires off the most activity during this restorative phase. When the body is away, the brain then comes out to play. Take the time just prior to sleeping to relax. We still need to fulfill our interpersonal needs. Conscious breathing, meditation, affirmations, and simple relaxation are great ways to take the brain down from the activity of the day.

Conscious breathing is simply being aware of your breathing. Taking what would otherwise be a subconscious act and focusing all of your attention to it. Establish a baseline knowledge of your breathing. Do you usually breathe fast? Does inhalation happen at the same rate of exhalation? Does your chest rise? Can you hear your breathing?

Breathing that is audible, by design is flawed. The noise you hear as you breathe is the byproduct of an obstacle in the upper respiratory system. As you work through airway optimization you should be able to get to quiet breathing. Those quiet breaths can be varied as you take conscious control. There are four excellent breathwork exercises that I always share and vary through my own daily conscious mediation.

- Rhythmic breathing: play your favorite song on a personal device. Have your breath dance to the music as it plays. Find the rhythm of the song and breathe along. Let the rhythm flow through your nostrils, dance around your lungs, and flow back out through your nostrils.
- Detox breathing: become conscious of your breathing and take control of your inhalation and breath for a count of four seconds. Exhale and release the waste of the air, deeply to a count of six seconds. Repeat for a minimum of one minute.
- Box breathing: take in an inhale for four seconds, then hold that breath for four seconds. Exhale for four seconds, then hold that breath for four seconds. Repeat for a minimum of one minute.

- Diaphragmatic breathing: start with an inhale and fill your belly with air, be mindful of expansion. As you exhale, let the air escape the belly and flow back out through your nostrils. Do not allow your chest or shoulders to rise and fall as you are breathing. All movement should be in the belly. Repeat for a minimum of one minute.

These may be paired with mantras or affirmations, or positive phrases, to guide you into a better night. Our minds thrive on the messages given and internalized. If you believe it, you will achieve it. Very cliché, but also very true. Every thought that you have – be it defeating, self-deprecating, empowering, or inspiring – will create your mental foreshadowing and impact the outcomes of all things you put forward.

This becomes the most obvious if you do sales work. Take, for example, my time in clinical dental hygiene. Not your average sales job, but highly focused on sales and not where you would imagine. The dentist that is over-diagnosing cavities is a rare occurrence. It is, however, the little things like the extra diagnostic tests and fluoride offers that comprise the sales process.

Contrary to popular belief, there are dental hygienists that do not believe in fluoride. They are adamantly opposed for reasons unknown to me. I am not one of those and feel conversely very positive about it. I have never had a cavity in my life. I have all 32 teeth in my mouth and am an average brusher. I use an electric toothbrush and floss when I feel like it. So, my oral hygiene is not the savior of my teeth. As a current vegan, I would also say my diet is not preventing cavities. Fluoride is my sole contributor to the lack of decay. Needless to say, with that message internalized deeply within me, I have no qualms selling it at the end of a cleaning. I genuinely feel that everyone should have it. (I also would like to add that I do not harass my patients about flossing, because I can give or take that personally. No contradictions here.)

Selling fluoride is easy, and I am willing to do so without much prodding of upper management. However, I have yet to personally perform an oral cancer screening that comes back positive. I have colleagues with stories about the supplemental tests saving the lives of one or two people they have encountered with positive results. It is never a story about helping numerous people, it is always the greater minority of people. So, while yes, I value the importance of early detection, I can also acknowledge that for the majority, it is unnecessary. Selling early oral cancer detection tests I find to be drawing a personal line. My internal message has that set to no.

These internal messages and beliefs are powerful and influence daily behavior whether obvious or not. We have to silence the little voice that works against you to fill the mind with positive thoughts to fulfill our esteem needs. This is critical before bed as the subconscious mind takes over during REM and the brain stores all the day's information. Those thoughts you filled the mind with will be deposited in the memory banks. Are those last thoughts you had inspiring or deprecating?

Download my 36-card set of affirmations to use or display throughout the day and to reflect on during this relaxation period at https://bit.ly/pbmaffirm.

Empowering your mindset prior to falling asleep will encourage subconscious confidence and favorable dreaming. Since every morning is dependent on the quality of sleep you had the night before, relaxation sets an encouraging tone for your productive tomorrow.

Efficiency

"I knew I could control one thing, and that is my time and my hours and my effort and my efficiency" -Ryan Seacrest

A great night of sleep usually ends with you awaking naturally and feeling reasonably refreshed. Reasonable refreshment is not jumping out of the bed and heading straight to work. You should rise and be able to reflect either on a good dream or just feeling well. However, do not linger long in the dark. Turn down your body's melatonin production with exposure to natural light. Open the blinds, pull back the curtain, step out onto the porch, or use artificial blue light eliminating light bulbs.

Sunlight is related to the production of the hormone serotonin. Commonly known for antidepressant ability, this natural mood and focus enhancer, starts your day off effectively. Get your morning routine started shortly after to make good use of this boost.

True restoration through C.A.R.E. leads to optimal sleep, which in turn, provides you with the energy and mental aptitude necessary for peak productivity. We need to take it up a notch for self-actualization. To be successful, we established a required combination of disciplined choices and habits. To accomplish your goals and get the most out of your day will require that same level of commitment.

Preplanning your day and being accountable for the results of that day keeps you on the productivity path long term. Let's be real, this book is not called "Done." There is a finality to the word done. You can have a goal and complete it to be done; however, long term goals are things you consider your accomplishments. Finally getting through a marathon you practiced a year for, working with big clients and landing the promotion you longed for or losing the 30 pounds you struggled with are all celebratory successes. Sure, you can celebrate smaller goals like making it through the day on only one coffee, finally leaving work on time, or maintaining the will power to say no to dessert, but consider those things done, not accomplished.

When planning your predictable day, keep it 100 with expectations. Do not over-plan your day to make it unrealistic to complete. Plan tasks that will bring you closer to your goals but not unrealistic to complete. Start with making a list of what needs to get done to reach the end. When writing this book, I gave myself 30 days and a daily goal of five pages a day. You may not reach your goal daily, but every step in the right direction is still progress. Make it realistic and achievable.

Having your plan and keeping your plan are two different things. To keep yourself on track, it helps to be accountable. Recruit or hire someone to have your back. Remember that we still need to achieve our social and personal esteem levels to reach self-actualization. Consider asking a friend, colleague, acquaintance, or family member to be your accountability partner. Alternatively, you can hire an accountability coach with professional experience to walk the path with you. Essentially, someone who is willing to encourage the progress you make or push you to get back on track when things go awry. Honesty is the key, so this should be someone you are comfortable being honest with.

Check-in daily with three messages.

- ***Rise and Shine*** – You're up and ready to go after a great night of restorative sleep. With this message you want to briefly recap your morning routine and set the intention for the day. Lead with the amount of sleep you got, how refreshed you feel or any dreams you remember. Next, announce your intentions or the daily affirmation that will get you through. Example: "Good Morning! I slept seven hours and woke up before my alarm! Feeling good going into the day with today's affirmation: 'I am unbreakable.' "

- ***Into the Grind*** – Once you have fully immersed yourself into your daily grind, share your progress. This message is helpful to send after a small achievement in the day. Everyone loves good news, so to be the bearer of said news, as an added testament to your overall growth. Keep it brief and positive. Example: "Just had lunch and I am unbreakable! Finished my presentation three days early!"
    - If you have no good news to share, then please still share. Maintain accountability while retaining compassion and empathy for yourself. The greatest self-love is that of which you continue to keep for yourself when you least want to. You are worthy of compassion even in your worst moments. Grant yourself this ultimate honor and you will never regret it. Example: "Rough morning. The meeting ran late, and I forgot my lunch at home. However, I am unbreakable! I am going to make some

progress on the presentation this
afternoon, even if I have to stay a little
later."

- *C.A.R.E. Confirmation* – Even our most productive days have an ending. We are not the pink battery bunny that keeps going. So, end the day with your accountability partner giving them a brief summary of any progress and that your C.A.R.E. routine is done. This is a good moment to reflect on where you are and begin planning the next day. Example: "Today was fair, I did most of the presentation. Planning on finishing it tomorrow. I am unbreakable! CARE done! Good night."

In short, take C.A.R.E. and take charge. Be consistent with bedtime, manage your airway and relax for optimal restoration. Remember that every good day starts with a good sleep the night prior. Wake feeling refreshed, start up the serotonin and remain accountable.

"Now you know, and knowing is half the battle." - G.I. Joe

Understanding the C.A.R.E. process and implementing it into your daily routine are two different things. When working with clients as a myofunctional therapist, I first start with asking about goals. What are the client's goals, and how can I best help them achieve it? In some cases, their ideas about what myofunctional therapy can help them accomplish are not realistic. Then we consider what they can achieve and if it is in alignment with my skills.

With the C.A.R.E. process, it is no different. Step 1 is to establish what your goals are for the entire process. Will this be a year-long journey of accomplishment, or does it have a shorter duration? What are the micro-goals or achievements that need to be done along the way? What is the timeline for each step to be completed?

These should be thought out in preparation, well before you begin. Start with your main objective by answering this question: if you overcame your biggest problem how would life change? For example, if your biggest problem is wanting to make a change in your career, the main objective would be to have fulfillment at work by becoming a(n) <u>career title here</u>. The main objective, in this case, is measurable by not just the achievement of the position, but also by esteem needs being met.

To complete the main objective or primary goal, there are tasks that need to happen first. To change a career returning to school, obtaining a certification, getting an internship or apprenticeship, advancing within the company, or getting hired at a new company would need to preface that accomplishment. Just like pants must be put on one leg at a time, accomplishment comes one step at a time. Each of these is considered a sub-goal. I suggest when filling out the C.A.R.E. worksheet, on page 105, to have at least three sub-goals but no more than five. Write them down in linear order and set a realistic timeframe for completion for each one. The sum of which will give you your accomplished schedule. Whether long or short in duration, the process aims to utilize your goal as motivation while obtaining true restoration for peak productivity, which enables you to reach the main objective.

The next step is to consider how to personalize your consistency, airway management, relaxation, and efficiency course of action. Consistency planning takes into account your current routine and how to best revise it to optimize it. Easy enough to replicate daily and integrate into the lifestyle. Simple things like dinner and personal hygiene are obvious but consider things that may help discern a transition to bedtime; such as a warm bath, reading a book, quality time with a spouse or family member, working on a side hustle, enjoying a massage, or sitting by candlelight to watch the sun set with a glass of wine. What small incorporation can you commit to? Make a list of possibilities and consider the time you have between dinner and bed prior to deciding. This routine is not final, by any means; however, refrain from making changes without a few weeks of trial.

Airway management will be the most difficult to plan. Nasal hygiene is the wisest starting point. Aromatherapy, nasal spray, saline rinse, nasal strip, and/or nasal dilators can be used together in a routine or independently. If you have no experience with any of the aforementioned, begin with a nasal saline spray. Blow the nose to clear the path, then insert the nozzle of the spray into a nostril and spray on inhale. Always follow the directions on the packaging, but this method has worked on my family and clients with no adverse reactions. Once you become accustomed to the nasal spray, consider using a dilator or strip to hold open the nose during sleep.

Tracking your sleep during the initial weeks will be helpful in determining what works. Use an app or smart device for at least one week to gauge the average. The apps and devices are not (with great emphasis on NOT) a substitute for a professional sleep study. The data collected measures what the device can interpret based on several factors, such as heart rate and movement. Electronics are unable to distinguish between restless sleep and movement after laying idle on the couch for an hour. Use the data wisely, but also keep track of any common signs of a sleep disorder.

Common Signs of a Sleep Disorder

Daytime sleepiness	Difficulty falling asleep
Difficulty staying asleep	Irritability or mood swings
Strong urge to nap	Clenching or Grinding
Loud snoring	Poor concentration
Bedwetting	Sleep Walking

Consult a sleep physician, pulmonologist, otolaryngologist, or your primary physician if you see irregular results during self-monitoring. There are also sleep dentists that can offer good insight and may be more accessible. These dentists use devices that make permanent or temporary adjustments to the jaws, allowing more airway space. They screen and assess for sleep breathing disorders. Not all dentists are airway friendly or fully knowledgeable, find a list of trusted professionals on any of these internet directories:

- Foundation for Airway Health – Airway Advocates
  - www.airwayhealth.org
- American Academy of Dental Sleep Medicine
  - www.aadsm.org
- American Academy of Physiological Medicine and Dentistry – Professional Directory

- ○ www.aapmd.org
- The Breathe Institute – Ambassadors Directory
  - ○ www.thebreatheinstitute.com

Just in case you missed this in the last chapter, myofunctional therapy can be a life-changer when it comes to airway management. I do have an obvious bias, however, that does not discount the effectiveness. With or without a known sleep disorder, eliminating dysfunction of the mouth and face will set you up for optimized sleep.

On the C.A.R.E. worksheet, write down the contact information of local sleep and dental professionals. Whether you use the information or not, the purpose is convenience. Then check off your preferences for nasal hygiene. Nasal hygiene should be integrated into your daily routine.

Relaxation can be done in conjunction with airway management. Aromatherapy diffusion in a room, while you are meditating can be a beautiful combination of opening the nostrils, decongestion, and pacification. Make a short-list of practical things you could do to ease yourself into bed. The concept of mediation can be anxiety-producing, be assured that there are no limits to relaxing possibilities. Reading, journaling, listening to soft music or white noise are all viable alternatives. List some options on your C.A.R.E. worksheet and experiment for a few days with each before you determine what the long-term plan will be.

Efficiency is often the easiest to plan and the most difficult to fulfill. Note what you would like to do within the first few minutes of walking to get that circadian rhythm going. Opening the blinds, pulling back the curtain, stepping out onto a porch, turning on some lights, or hoping straight into a shower. Get the ball rolling and the day started. How will you capitalize on your restored body's new energy surge?

Accountability will be key for the check-in messages. Your partner can be anyone you can rely on to not just receive your messages, but to respond as needed to support you. Write down the names and information of two possible partners.

On your daily C.A.R.E. journal entries, determine the plan for the day and consider what sub-goal you plan to achieve in the near future. The goal should be written down daily. The more you write it, read it, and repeat it, the more likely you are to achieve it. As your day progresses write down either a brief summary of the check-in messages or the full text. Keep track of your daily progress and write down the goal for the following day on the next page. Many times the goal may be the same, do not feel discouraged, all steps forward is progress.

In the preliminary days of working this program with my clients, I had them consider similar aspects to arrive at our C.A.R.E. plan towards our larger goal of orofacial health or development. Three categories of goals emerged: health, family, and business. I have one of each type that I want to present to you to help you realize how personal and flexible it can be.

Productivity Profile: Client A
C.A.R.E. Case – Family

Client A made her goal balancing life with grace. Not a measurable goal from an outside perspective. However, her sub-goals were defined well. Have enough energy to wake up before her kids without feeling tired, getting home on time daily to meet the school bus, and making dinner six out of seven nights a week.

A made self-contact, no referral from medical or dental providers. Concerned about a tongue tie due to information she read on social media, she reached out for more information on the process. She did have a tongue tie as well as low tongue resting posture, open bite, forward head posture, and cranial nerve asymmetries in V, VII, and XII.

Weeks 1-4

C- Consistent routine at bedtime, led by client current routine with minor adjustments. Get kids in bed, watch one television show, take a shower, brush, and floss to be completed by 10:30pm.

A – Myofunctional therapy sessions one time weekly with a focus on cranial nerve balancing. Nasal hygiene routine involves saline rinse followed by aromatherapy inhaler. Practice exercises two times daily, once before bed.

R – Quiet reflection and journaling of the day's events.

E – Establish an accountability partner and check in with three daily messages. Sub-goal to focus on with messaging: waking refreshed and before the kids. 6-week timeline for goal achievement.

Weeks 5-8

C – Consistent routine at bedtime to be maintained. The client held routine but often with completion at 11:00pm. Shower removed from nighttime to morning at the client's discretion to reclaim 30 minutes deficit.

A – The client prepared for and received tongue-tie release. Myofunctional therapy put on hold for one week during active wound management and resumed at week 6. Week 8 client consulted with a dentist for a removable appliance.

R – The client enjoys this part of the process most and chooses to extend the journaling process.

E – Accountability partner established at week four. Sub-goal achieved at week seven. A new sub-goal of getting home on time daily has a -week timeline. A few weeks of job interviews were to proceed to accommodate the goal and end the workday earlier.

Weeks 9-12

C – Consistent routine at bedtime moved back to 11:00pm. The client waking refreshed after an average of six hours of sleep. Routine adjusted to allow for refreshment and optimize evening routine time.

A – Myofunctional therapy sessions rounding out into habituation as the client establishes exercises into daily activities and functions. The appliance is worn daily and consistent. Open bite closed and tongue postured up at rest. The client completed myofunctional program at week 12.

R – The client added yoga and meditation to relaxation. 1-hour process of quiet reflection with journaling minimized to 10 minutes routine.

E – Accountability partner communication consistent. New job consists of work from home. New sub-goal to make dinner six out of seven evenings a week started prior to previous goal completion. 4-week timeline to completion.

3-Month Check-In

The client maintained C.A.R.E. process since program completion. The appliance is creating forward growth of the upper arch as well as width. Open bite, low tongue posture, and cranial nerve asymmetries all eliminated and new habits retained. Personal goal accomplished to client satisfaction as she is home daily to wake her children and greet them after school. Meals are homemade six nights a week and energy levels are steady throughout the day. Accountability checks ceased once the client felt that goals were complete. Efficiency replaced with waking to sun exposure with breakfast on an enclosed porch.

<h2 style="text-align:center">Productivity Profile: Client B
C.A.R.E. Case – Health</h2>

Referred by a Naturopathic Physician due to persistent mouth breathing and strong gag reflex. At 17 years old, client B, presented with a history of asthma, tonsil removal, crooked teeth, and TMJ pain on wide opening. His evaluation found a tongue thrust swallow, weak soft palate lift, and cranial nerve asymmetry in V, VII, IX, X, XI, and XII. Goals, as determined by parents, are to achieve optimal health and eliminate pain by 18th birthday. I had parents define optimal health to be two or less colds per year and no asthma attacks. Sub goals are to eliminate pain in the jaw, sleep with mouth closed, and complete orthodontic treatment.

Weeks 1-5

C – Consistent bedtime routine made collaboratively with referring doctor. Dinner to be gluten and dairy-free daily, hot water bath for therapeutic steam for 20 mins, followed by a shower, and brushing.

A – Myofunctional therapy sessions bi-weekly for the first three weeks for cranial nerve work to be established. Prescribed myofunctional exercises to be done three times daily, once prior to bedtime nasal hygiene. Nasal hygiene routine with xylitol nasal rinse and nasal dilator insertion.

R – Relaxation routine to be with conscious breathing mediation, at the client's request.

E – Establish note file in smartphone with prewritten C.A.R.E. check-in text messages to send parents after each myofunctional exercise practice session. Elimination of pain in jaw estimated completion time of six weeks.

Weeks 6-11

C – Bedtime routine unchanged. The client is relatively consistent and struggles with avoiding gluten and dairy.

A – Myofunctional therapy sessions once weekly with a focus on gag desensitizing and soft palate lift strengthening. Prescribed exercises and nasal hygiene to remain as before.

R – The client elects to modify relaxation to exclude conscious breathing and insert music during meditation. Reverted to conscious breathing as a part of my therapy during week eight.

E – Check-in messages are done consistently. Jaw pain reduced but not eliminated. The timeline on goals changed to 10 weeks. During week nine client sleeping daily with mouth closed.

Weeks 12-15

C – More consistent with diet modifications. A bedtime routine is decidedly permanent. Sleeping on average for eight hours and waking up without an alarm, feeling rested. Starts the day by opening the curtains.

A - Myofunctional therapy sessions rounding out into habituation as The client establishes exercises into daily activities and functions. Nasal dilator exchanged for nasal strips. The client completed myofunctional program at week 15. Recommended parents to a dental provider of an appliance for mandibular advancement, opted for traditional braces.

R – The client still conscious breathing for relaxation. The client began journaling during week 13.

E – Check-in messages done with parents until week 12, then done with a girlfriend. Jaw pain eliminated unless the client has a maximum opening. Orthodontist started treatment during week 14. The goal of braces completion in two years.

4-Month Check-In

C.A.R.E. process maintained since program completion. Mouth breathing eliminated and gag reflex normalized. The last asthma attack nine months prior, reduced congestion over the winter season during the program, and energy levels improved. Cranial nerves balanced and thrust swallow reduced. The client feeling overall healthier and notices better sleep and more energy. The referring physician sent the client for sleep study post-program, with results showing no signs of apnea.

Productivity Profile: Client C and me
C.A.R.E. Case – Business

Client C made self-contact due to curiosity after a friend had a child who completed myofunctional therapy. The client presented with few issues common to myofunctional cases, i.e. improper oral posture, tongue tie, and mouth breathing. However, he reported poor sleep and feeling perpetually tired. As a vice president in a corporation, he wanted a simple program with rapid results in a short time. (No pressure) This is a pure C.A.R.E. case with little myofunctional therapy and more dynamic work through breathwork and mindset coaching. Initial evaluation found allergic shiners, class II dental occlusion, and cranial nerve asymmetry in CN VIII and X. Goals are to establish a sleep routine for optimal sleep and complete structured report for board members in 30 days.

Weeks 1-2

C – Boundaries set in the beginning. Client to establish a bedtime routine based on realistic expectations of leaving work. The client often works until 11PM and arrives home 40 minutes later to hop into bed and sleep. The client resistant to leaving work early, an in-bed goal to be 12:30 AM. Late-night routines will not include dinner because sleep is altered if digestion is happening actively during sleep. Avoid eating less than two hours before sleep. Upon arrival, the client will prepare lunch for the next day and read a book in the massage chair. The client very cooperative and routinely performed daily.

A – Week 1 with a focus on cranial nerve balancing and breathwork. The client to perform nasal hygiene with a saline rinse. Breathwork focuses on two exercises with the client to perform immediately after the nasal hygiene routine and during relaxation.

R – The client does not enjoy any quiet mediation and very resistant. Relaxation occurs through laying in bed with focus conscious breathing.

E- The client makes no attempt to have an accountability partner. I elect to join his C.A.R.E. journey and be his partner with a personal goal to complete this book by the end of the journey. Week two check-in messages begin coming in routinely. Reports less lethargy during the day but still wakes to feel unrefreshed. Goal to establish a sleep routine set for completion in four weeks, concurrently set with the goal to complete board report.

Week 3-4

C – The client started to leave work at 10:30 to have more time for book consumption during a bedtime routine. Consistent with a bedtime routine. I personally established a bedtime routine of self-Reiki, writing, and brushing.

A – Breathwork moved to the client choice of one exercise after nasal hygiene. The client came across the concept of taping. Encouraged the client to try during the daytime slowly before trying bedtime. In practice, I do not advise mouth taping, especially without a medical clearance that it would be safe for the client. The client chooses to try for one week.

R – Relaxation still occurring in bed with conscious breathing. The client finds that conscious breathing is happening for a shorter duration. Falling asleep at earlier periods during relaxation. Encouraged to continue and start 5-10 minutes earlier.

E – Check-in texts are consistent. The client reporting feeling more refreshed and waking prior to alarm daily. Completed report two days early and focused on finishing the program and getting settled into a routine to complete a goal of established sleep routine in the next two weeks. My check-in texts fueled the positivity and progress of the client's progress. Book has 30 pages and goal to complete extended to week six.

Weeks 5-6

C – Bedtime routine established. Leaving work at 10:30 PM and arriving home around 11:15PM. Sleeping on average five hours a night and reports waking up refreshed.

A – The client enjoyed mouth tapping but only committing to it for three days a week. Daily breathwork and conscious breathing after nasal hygiene routine. Reports waking with mouth closed at night and sleep tracker is recording less snoring.

R – Relaxation for seven minutes in bed, client content with results for sleep initiation.

E – The client well settled into a goal and feeling more energetic. Ended program with a gym routine early every morning for efficiency. Goals completed earlier than anticipated and client working on C.A.R.E. journal for next work goal. I completed this book in my 6-week timeline.

3-Month Check-In

The client enjoys the structure of the daily routine and has been consistent in self-guidance since. Sleeping on average five hours every night and no longer taping. Cranial nerve symmetry present and bags under eyes no longer present. Referred client to an orthodontist for consultation due to malocclusion, however, the client did not pursue any further.

"Do the best you can until you know better. Then when you know better do better." – Maya Angelou

You have made it to the crossroad. The junction between dysfunction and satisfaction. At this point you have a solid understanding of the impact of restorative sleep on productive ability. Your brain works hard for you during the day, fuels during sleep, and is prepped to keep you going. What you do with this information is now on you. Motivation without determination is merely a dream.

It is my hope that this book will serve as encouragement. This is halftime in the locker room. The team is down, but the game is not over. As a player you have to stay focused on the goal, and as a coach I have to remind you why we play. A firm nudge towards self-actualization. Though reaching that mountain peak may seem scary, the view from the peak is a million times greater than the gaze from below. The previous pages are your permanent reminder that you are capable of identifying and tackling barriers, be they personal or physical.

Re-read when necessary to gain clarity on aspects that resonated with you. Ask for help. There is no shame is getting help. Few ever do hike alone. On the ascent you may need a helping hand. Contact specialists near you or reach out to me and my team. We will help plan and structure your personalized plan.

Whether you start solo or with assistance the key is getting started. Practice will make perfect. The C.A.R.E. plan you start with may be different than that which will be a permanent fixture. You will evolve during this process and have new desires. Dive deep into those and embrace the change.

At our core, we are human. Simple with basic biological needs of air, food and water. The steppingstone to success is founded strongly on the fulfillment of those needs. How we intake air and food will impact sleep and health. The way you breathe matters. Prioritize the optimization of the bare necessities and you will glide into success.

Never underestimate the work involved in achieving long term retention of these new habits. Airway management is a process of relearning habits that have been present for most of your life. They will not go away overnight. Your journey of deprogramming will be different than others. It may be longer and harder, or quicker and shorter. The process to self-actualization is equally as personal as sleep.

Life is too short to do anything short of making yourself happy. Whether personal or physical barriers to that happiness exist, there is no better time to eliminate them. Remember that the formula begins with function. When dysfunction is present, peak productivity is impossible. The notorious examples of success with little sleep are not freaks of nature. They have the tools to win the rat race of life and are optimizing every waking hour to continue to achieve more. You can reach this level of accomplished.

Everyone can use a little care, which is why C.A.R.E. is for everyone.

Resources

As a final support to your growth on your journey to accomplished, I want to leave you with resources. The first resources I want to mention are ones that I provide for free. Visit www.themyospot.com to learn more about airway disorders, options, fast facts, and myofunctional therapy services. There are also many great supplemental reading posts on our blog: www.airwaymatters.blog

Next, is yet another personal invitation to join one of our Accomplished Network Facebook groups and communities. Divided into three key groups of focus goals. Join one or all to find similarly motivated people. These communities are there to support you in completing your C.A.R.E. worksheet, journal, finding an accountability partner, and motivation.

CARE Family: **facebook.com/groups/accomplishedfamily**

CARE Health: **facebook.com/groups/accomplishedhealth**

CARE Business: **facebook.com/groups/accomplishwork**

There's no way I would leave you without a way to track your progress. The C.A.R.E. journal can be found on Amazon for purchase, or see the last few pages of this book for a start.

Finally, support your knowledge through other outlets by diving into some other airway focused books I love:

Jaws by Dr. Sandra Kahn

Tongue Tied by Dr. Richard Baxter et al.

Six Foot Tiger, Three Foot Cage by Dr. Felix Liao

The Dental Diet by Dr. Steven Lin

GASP Airway Health: The Hidden Path To Wellness by Dr. Michael Gelb and Dr. Howard Hindin

Sleep, Interrupted by Dr. Steven Y Park

C.A.R.E.

My accomplishment goal:

____

Goal completion date: _____/_____/_____

<u>Steps to complete</u>

Sub achievement:_________________________________

Timeline to achieve: _______ weeks/months

Sub achievement: _________________________________

Timeline to achieve: _______ weeks/months

Sub achievement: _________________________________

Timeline to achieve: _______ weeks/months

Sub achievement: _________________________________

Timeline to achieve: _______ weeks/months

Sub achievement: _________________________________

Timeline to achieve: _______ weeks/months

C.A.R.E. Worksheet

Consistent Planning

Current Routine:

____

____

I can add/remove:

____

____

Desired Bedtime:

______:______AM/PM

Determined Routine:

____

____

Airway Management Planning

Nasal hygiene:

☐ Saline Rinse ☐ Aromatherapy

☐ Nasal Spray ☐ Nasal Strip

☐ Nasal Dilator

Myofunctional Therapist-

____

Website/Address:

____

Phone Number:

____

Relaxation Planning

I feel most relaxed when:

____

____

Before bed I will relax by:

____

____

____

Alternate relaxation ideas:

____

____

Efficient Planning

My alarm is set for:

______:______ AM/PM

When I wake up I will immediately

____

____

____

My accountability partner(s):

Name:_______________________

Number:_______________________

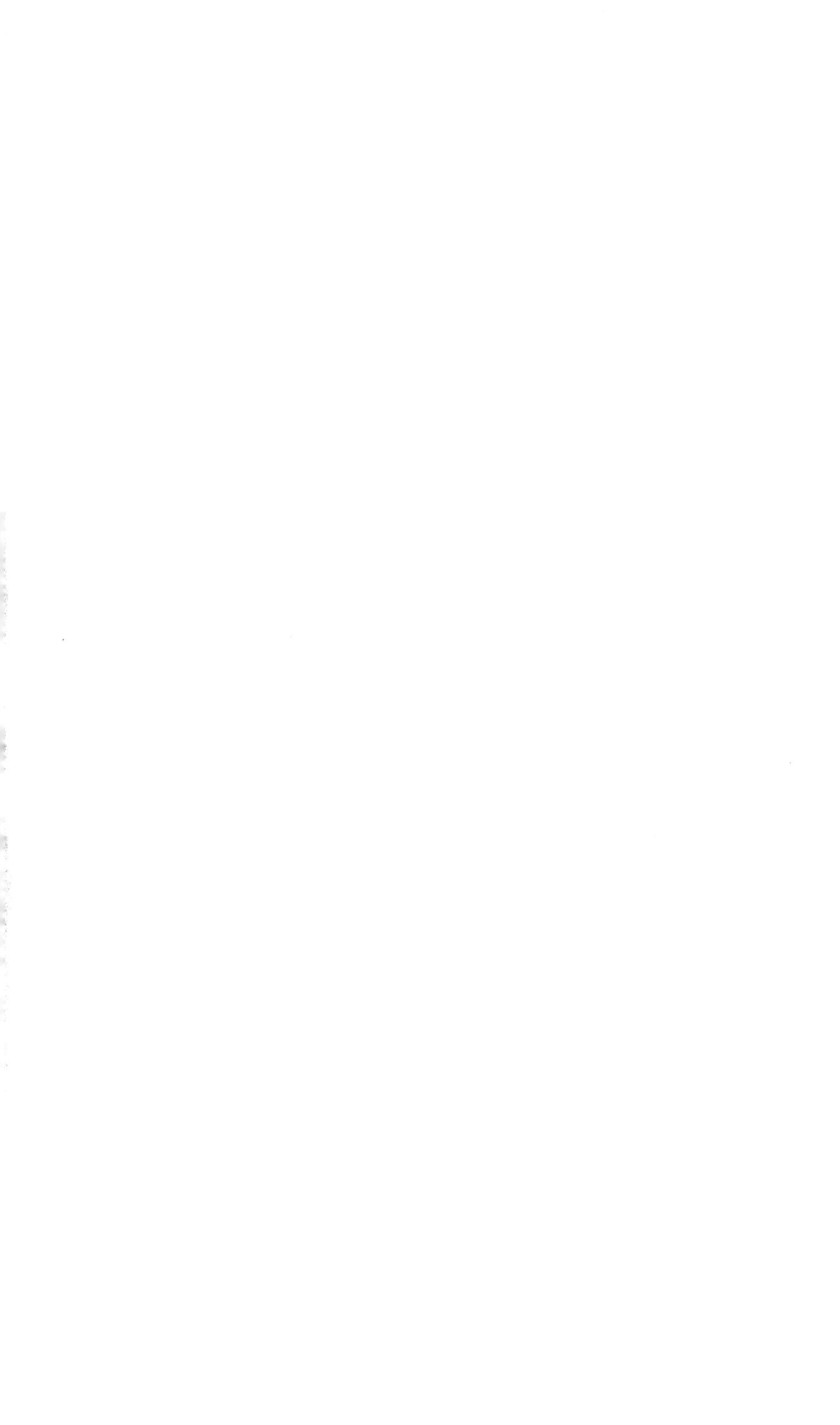